Treating Substance Use Disorders
With Adaptive Continuing Care

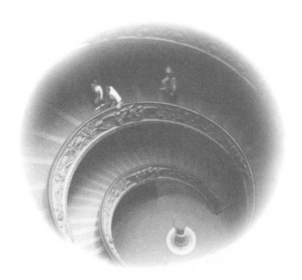

Treating Substance Use Disorders
With Adaptive Continuing Care

JAMES R. McKAY

American Psychological Association • *Washington, DC*

Published by
American Psychological Association
750 First Street, NE
Washington, DC 20002
www.apa.org

To order
APA Order Department
P.O. Box 92984
Washington, DC 20090-2984
Tel: (800) 374-2721; Direct: (202) 336-5510
Fax: (202) 336-5502; TDD/TTY: (202) 336-6123
Online: www.apa.org/books/
E-mail: order@apa.org

In the U.K., Europe, Africa, and the Middle East, copies may be ordered from
American Psychological Association
3 Henrietta Street
Covent Garden, London
WC2E 8LU England

Typeset in Goudy by Stephen McDougal, Mechanicsville, MD

Printer: Maple-Vail Books, York, PA
Cover Designer: Naylor Design, Washington, DC
Technical/Production Editor: Devon Bourexis

Library of Congress Cataloging-in-Publication Data

McKay, James R.
   Treating substance use disorders with adaptive continuing care / James R. McKay. — 1st ed.
      p. cm.
   Includes bibliographical references.
   ISBN-13: 978-1-4338-0459-5
   ISBN-10: 1-4338-0459-X
   1. Substance abuse—Psychological aspects. 2. Substance abuse—Treatment. I. Title.

   HV4998.M45 2009
   616.86'06—dc22   2008054513

British Library Cataloguing-in-Publication Data
A CIP record is available from the British Library.

Printed in the United States of America
First Edition

This book is dedicated to Mike Bodeen, Jay McGrath, and Jim Vinton, with deep appreciation for their honesty, generosity, and encouragement.

CONTENTS

ACKNOWLEDGMENTS

One of the most enjoyable aspects of doing addiction treatment research has been the wonderful mentors and colleagues I have had over the years, who have deeply influenced my thinking about continuing care and helped facilitate the work I have done. I am particularly grateful for my collaborations and discussions with Steve Maisto, Tom McLellan, Jon Morgenstern, and Kevin Lynch. I have also had the pleasure of working on a number of projects with gifted and generous investigators from the University of Pennsylvania and other institutions, including Arthur Alterman, John Cacciola, Kathy Carroll, Linda Collins, Mike Dennis, John Finney, Mike French, Keith Humphreys, Dan Kivlahan, Dick Longabaugh, David Mark, Susan Murphy, Chuck O'Brien, Tim O'Farrell, Dave Oslin, Helen Pettinati, Don Shepard, Debbie Van Horn, and Connie Weisner. Most of the ideas presented in this book are in some way an outgrowth of conversations with the individuals mentioned here.

I am also indebted to my dedicated and highly skilled research staff, which has included several project coordinators—Donna Coviello, Megan Ivey, Janelle Koppenhaver, Rebecca Morrison, Sara Ratichek, and Kathleen Ward—as well as numerous research technicians and counselors. Without these individuals, the work described in this book would not have been completed, nor would the book itself have been written.

Funding for my work has been provided by the National Institute on Alcohol Abuse and Alcoholism and the National Institute on Drug Abuse. I am grateful for the continuous support received from both institutes, as well as the interest that Debra Grossman, Bob Huebner, Cherry Lowman, Lisa Onken, Harold Perl, Cecelia Spitznas, Mark Willenbring, and other staff members have shown in our work on continuing care and adaptive treatments.

My wife, Rachel, and my daughters, Madeline and Nina, also deserve considerable thanks for supporting my efforts to complete this book. This is especially the case because my initial plans to write this book during a sabbatical from the University of Pennsylvania were nixed when I accepted an additional position at the Philadelphia Veterans Affairs Medical Center. So, in time-honored fashion, much of this book was completed in the evenings and on weekends. In addition, Rachel's considerable clinical skill and keen observations, so clearly apparent in our conversations about treatment over more than 20 years, have had a major influence on my thinking about how to help people with substance use disorders.

The staff at the American Psychological Association has been most helpful in bringing this project along through each step of the process. I would like to thank the acquisition editors, Lansing Hays and Susan Reynolds, the development editor, Beth Hatch, and the production editor, Devon Bourexis, for their encouragement, support, and suggestions regarding revisions. I also thank Ed Meidenbauer and three anonymous reviewers, for their extensive feedback on earlier drafts of the manuscript, and Lauren Skalina, for help with literature reviews and references.

Finally, I'm particularly grateful to the more than 2,000 individuals from publicly funded addiction treatment programs and the Veterans Affairs Medical Center in Philadelphia who have participated in the studies performed by my group over the past 16 years. I also thank the directors and treatment staff from these programs, who have been strongly supportive of our work.

I

THE CASE FOR
CONTINUING CARE IN
ADDICTION TREATMENT

1

INTRODUCTION

Alcohol and drug abuse and dependence are among the more common debilitating health problems in the United States, with approximately 9% of the population meeting *Diagnostic and Statistical Manual of Mental Disorders* (*DSM–IV*; 4th ed.; American Psychiatric Association, 1994) diagnostic criteria for an alcohol or drug use disorder in the prior 12 months (Grant et al., 2004). Moreover, they are among the most costly. Recent estimates of the costs of various medical disorders indicate that the economic cost of alcohol and drug use disorders is approximately $185 and $180 billion per year, respectively. This means that the cost of alcohol use disorders alone is as great as that of heart disease ($183 billion/year) and more than Alzheimer's disease and other dementias ($100 billion), obesity ($99 billion), diabetes ($98 billion), stroke ($43 billion), and HIV/AIDS ($29 billion; Office of National Drug Control Policy, 2004). Of course, these economic data do not begin to capture the suffering caused by addiction and the damage done to relationships with family and friends, as well as to others in the community.

Some individuals with substance use disorders are able to achieve sustained recoveries either on their own or after receiving a brief therapeutic intervention (Babor & Grant, 1992; L. C. Sobell, Sobell, Toneatto, & Leo, 1993). Others are able to stop drinking or drug use by attending self- or mutual-help programs such as Alcoholics Anonymous (AA; Humphreys, 2004).

However, many people with substance use disorders are unable to moderate or stop their use of alcohol or drugs through these methods and consequently end up in the formal treatment system. For these individuals, substance abuse is often a chronic disorder, characterized by periods of abstinence followed by eventual relapse and reentry into the treatment system (Hser, Longshore, & Anglin, 2007). Indeed, substance use disorders are increasingly seen as similar in course and outcome to chronic health problems such as diabetes, hypertension, and asthma (Dennis & Scott, 2007; McLellan, Lewis, O'Brien, & Kleber, 2000; Tims, Leukefeld, & Platt, 2001). Some investigators have used the terms *addiction careers* and *treatment careers* to capture the patterns of substance use and repeated treatment experiences observed in studies with follow-ups of a decade or more (Hser, Anglin, Grella, Longshore, & Prendergast, 1997; Hser et al., 2007).

To address the chronic nature of substance use disorders, the field of addiction treatment has increasingly focused on the development, implementation, and evaluation of *continuing care* interventions (McKay, 2005, 2006). These interventions are provided for some period of time after discharge from an initial, more intensive treatment experience. A typical example of a continuing care intervention is weekly group counseling after residential or intensive outpatient treatment. However, patients who enter residential or outpatient treatment after completing a brief detoxification intervention could be said to be in continuing care, as could patients engaged in general psychotherapy after the completion of addiction treatment.

At this point, there are a number of other terms in the addiction treatment field that imply or are in some way associated with the concept of continuing care (McKay, 2005). These include *aftercare, step-down care, stepped care, continuum of care,* and *disease management.* The differences between these terms are addressed later in this chapter and at various points in this book. However, *continuing care* and these related terms all describe service delivery mechanisms that are based on the belief that treatment for substance use disorders typically requires some phase of care beyond the initial acute care episode. Regardless of which terms are used to describe continuing care, the goals of the interventions tend to be relatively consistent. For example, most interventions stress the following:

- easing the transition from a more intensive to a less intensive form of treatment;
- facilitating reentry into the community, if the first phase of treatment involved residential or inpatient care;
- consolidating gains made in the initial phase of care;
- facilitating ongoing participation in self- and mutual-help programs;
- providing social support through group counseling;
- addressing relapse risks as they emerge;

- providing support for efforts to deal with co-occurring problems; and
- linking the patient to other sources of support in the community.

It has been widely believed that continuing care interventions that achieved these goals would lead to better extended management of addictive disorders, as indicated by lower relapse rates over time, less need for acute care episodes such as detoxification and emergency department visits, and better functioning in important life areas such as family and employment roles.

At this point, it is hard to find any clinicians or researchers working in the field of substance abuse treatment who will assert that patients with addictive disorders who enter the formal treatment system do not need continuing care (Dennis & Scott, 2007; Humphreys & Tucker, 2002; McLellan et al., 2000; Miller & Weisner, 2002). However, clinicians who treat addicted patients report that it is often difficult to deliver these interventions. This is frequently blamed on the lack of adequate funding for extended treatment. However, other severe impediments include high rates of dropout in the initial phase of treatment, before eligibility for continuing care, and lack of interest in continuing care among those who become eligible for it. For example, it is not uncommon for 50% or more of patients who begin a 4-week course of intensive outpatient treatment to drop out before completion and for another 50% to drop out before completion of a subsequent 12-week course of continuing care (McKay et al., 1997). In fact, recent data from a national survey of addiction treatment programs indicated that the median length of stay in outpatient and intensive outpatient programs was 76 and 46 days, respectively, with only 36% of admissions completing treatment (Substance Abuse and Mental Health Services Administration [SAMHSA], 2008). These high rates of relatively early dropout clearly limit the potential impact of efficacious continuing care interventions.[1]

CASE VIGNETTES

Three case vignettes are now presented as illustrations of the strengths and weaknesses of standard treatment for substance use disorders. The first vignette describes an individual who did well in a traditional, abstinence-oriented continuum of care that included detoxification, residential treatment, and outpatient continuing care, coupled with intensive participation

---

[1]It should be noted that some individuals who either never attend or dropout early from formal continuing care participate actively in self-help programs such as Alcoholics Anonymous and get considerable recovery support from these programs.

in self-help. The second and third vignettes, in contrast, are more representative of many of the patients we have seen in our clinics and practices.

The Motivated Patient With Support for Recovery

The young man, whom I refer to as William, was experiencing trouble with alcohol and drugs by the time he was 16. A strong student in prior grade levels, he barely avoided flunking most of his courses in his last years of high school. Disinterested in any further formal education, William did not bother applying to college and instead began working in retail sales positions. His problems with alcohol and drugs grew worse. Within a few years, he was engaging in morning drinking and often drank during his lunch breaks at work. William also did a fair amount of cocaine, usually in combination with alcohol.

By the time he was 22, William's family and friends were well aware that he had a serious problem because the evidence was unmistakable. William was also quite cognizant of the trouble his substance use was causing and was consumed by guilt and anxiety. He made frequent attempts to cut back, which sometimes worked, although not for long. After one particularly humiliating alcohol and drug binge, he contacted AA and began going to meetings. However, he continued to indulge in cocaine now and then, which soon enough led to relapse on alcohol.

Finally, at 24, William went into an inpatient detoxification program, following several major binges on alcohol and cocaine that had led to increasing pressure from friends and family to do something about his substance use problems. After a few days in the hospital, he was urged to go into a residential rehabilitation program but planned instead to return to work and take another stab at AA. William's employer, however, let him know with no uncertainty that he would not have a job if he did not go to rehab. The shame of losing a job trumped the embarrassment of going off to addiction treatment for a month, and away he went.

After completing a 28-day rehabilitation program, William returned home and did everything he had agreed to in his discharge plan. This included attending five or more AA meetings per week, getting an AA sponsor, and attending outpatient counseling. Over the first few months, William experienced the "honeymoon" period that is described in AA literature—his mood was good, he had no cravings or urges to use alcohol or drugs, and his anxiety and guilt had diminished considerably. At about the 3-month point, however, he experienced a return of strong cravings for cocaine. As the urges grew stronger, he found himself beginning to think seriously about using, despite how well his new life was going. At his daily AA meeting, he finally blurted out that he wanted to go out and use cocaine later that day and was seriously contemplating getting in his car and driving to his old dealer's house after the meeting. The urge suddenly disappeared and did not return. Over the next 7 years, he continued to attend AA regularly and maintained abstinence from alcohol and cocaine. Several years later, he returned briefly to drinking after not participating in AA for a while but was able to quickly stop by going to AA again.

This case vignette of an inspiring recovery is notable in several respects. First, William struggled at first to get sober, but after he entered treatment, he did well. Second, he had a positive response to what could be referred to as *standard treatment:* an inpatient rehabilitation program with a 12-step emphasis, followed by outpatient counseling and extended immersion in AA. Third, he did exactly what his treatment providers recommended at each turn, although a bit of leverage was required at a few points. In fact, he liked going to counseling and truly enjoyed participating in AA. Fourth, for the most part, he remained consistently abstinent and was bothered during those periods for only a relatively brief time with any serious thoughts about using again. When he did start drinking again, he was able to stop relatively easily by returning to self-help meetings. Finally, he had strong social support for abstinence, including friends who made it clear that he needed to get help, an employer who kept up the pressure for him to go into treatment, and AA members who were there for him when his commitment to abstinence wavered or went on a hiatus.

The Chronically Ambivalent Patient

Consider a second patient, whom I call Paul. He also abused alcohol and drugs as a teenager, although he graduated from high school in the top quarter of his class and was able to get into a good college. He continued to drink heavily in college and began to experience a number of negative consequences, such as blackouts, missed classes, and mediocre grades. After college, he was hired in a management position by a large corporation, and for a time, his drinking decreased. However, within 5 years, he found himself drinking more than he had planned with increasing frequency, in situations in which he had vowed to maintain better control "next time." After several work-related social events in which he embarrassed himself through inappropriate behavior and comments, he resolved to stop drinking. Unfortunately, this proved to be much more difficult than he had anticipated. Finally, in some desperation, he entered a detoxification program after progressing to drinking in the morning with some regularity following evenings of heavy drinking.

Like William, Paul was initially unwilling to consider going to a rehabilitation program after finishing detoxification. However, little pressure was put on him, and he persuaded the treatment staff and his employer that he would become active in AA. Paul did go to several self-help meetings, but he did not like the experience; he did not feel comfortable with the pressure to talk about himself, and he did not identify with others at the meetings. Furthermore, the emphasis on admitting powerlessness and turning his will over to a higher power was antithetical to his own philosophy of living. And, he had to admit, he really did not want to stop drinking entirely. So Paul stopped going to AA meetings after about 8 weeks of sporadic attendance. Within another month, he began drinking again, albeit less than before. Not surprisingly, however, he eventually began to experience nights of heavy drinking again, which ultimately progressed to binging frequently throughout the weekends.

Over the next 20 years, Paul cycled repeatedly between periods of controlled and uncontrolled alcohol use, interspersed with detoxifications and occasional treatment episodes. He never felt particularly comfortable with or good about treatment, and he continued to object to most of the basic teachings of 12-step programs. He usually did not complete outpatient treatment episodes, and when he did, almost never successfully negotiated the transition from one level of care to the next. At no point did Paul really participate in what might even remotely be seen as a continuum of care. There was no coordination between his successive treatment experiences. From Paul's perspective, the treatment system did not have anything to offer that was compatible with how he wanted to deal with his drinking problem.

The Patient With Barriers to Participation in Ongoing Treatment

Consider Joan, a third person with a history of substance abuse. Joan's experiences with the treatment system are also not uncommon. She is a single mother with two children, trying to reenter the workforce. She has had significant problems with cocaine for more than 10 years, which had led to legal complications and the threatened loss of custody of her children. When told she had to go into a rehabilitation program to maintain custody, she was only too willing to do so. She also made a good faith commitment to attend outpatient continuing care and self-help meetings but began to encounter multiple barriers in her effort to do so. It was difficult and embarrassing to tell a new employer that she had to leave work to attend addiction treatment. Child care was hard to come by, and expensive when it was available. The self-help meetings near her apartment were not a good fit for her, because they were attended largely by older men with whom she had little in common other than her addiction problems. Getting to other meetings in other neighborhoods by bus or subway was time-consuming. Trying to work and take care of her children took up a great deal of time and energy, and there was little left over for her efforts at recovery.

As time went by and these barriers did not lessen, Joan found that her commitment to attend treatment and AA began to diminish; it was just too demoralizing to try to make it to her sessions and meetings on a regular basis. Therefore, despite her real fears about what might happen, she gradually stopped participating in continuing care and self-help meetings.

LIMITATIONS OF STANDARD TREATMENT MODELS
IN THE ADDICTIONS

William's experience speaks volumes about how well our standard treatment system can work for individuals with alcohol and drug dependence. Unfortunately, his story is not typical of the majority of those who enter treatment for these disorders. Rather, people with substance use disorders are more likely to have experiences like Paul's and Joan's. For these patients, the continuum of care really is not a continuum at all. For example, most individuals who enter detoxification programs do not receive subsequent rehabilitation treatment, rates of sustained participation in outpatient treatment after residential treatment are low, more than half the patients who start treatment in outpatient programs drop out before completion, and rates of frequent participation in AA and other self-help programs plummet in the year after treatment (Humphreys, 2004; McKay, Merikle, Mulvaney, Weiss, & Koppenhaver, 2001; SAMHSA, 2008; Tonigan, Toscova, & Miller, 1996). For many people in our treatment system, addiction treatment therefore consists of repeated, isolated episodes of acute care with little or no coordination or follow-up.

The reality of our existing treatment system stands in sharp contrast to what has become a sea change in the way that most addiction treatment specialists and researchers think about the nature of addiction and the course of recovery. Specifically, there is now widespread acceptance that addiction is often a chronic problem characterized by increased vulnerability to relapse that can persist over many years, particularly among those who have entered the formal treatment system (Dennis & Scott, 2007; Humphreys & Tucker, 2002; McLellan et al., 2000). Clearly, this does not mean that addiction has all the same characteristics as other chronic medical disorders, such as hypertension, diabetes, or asthma. The course of these disorders can be significantly altered by changes in behavior, but in most cases, it is not possible to send them into remission by stopping a particular behavior, as is the case with alcohol or drug dependence. Rather, addiction looks like a chronic disorder in many cases because of the high probability of relapse early in recovery and the certainty of long-term heightened vulnerability to relapse.

The current emphasis in the field of addiction treatment on continuing care is a direct result of the conceptualization of substance use problems as chronic disorder for many who enter the formal treatment system. Most individuals involved with the provision of substance abuse treatment services, from counselors to program directors to state directors, think that it is important to provide continuing care services to patients who complete more intensive initial treatment episodes. As is discussed later in this book, in most cases this means weekly group counseling provided to patients who have completed residential treatment or an intensive outpatient program. For patients like William, this system can work remarkably well.

However, many patients are not like William. Studies have indicated that only 10% of those with substance use disorders get treatment in a given year (Institute of Medicine, 2001, 2006). Moreover, many people with substance use disorders who enter treatment do so with a great deal of ambivalence (DiClemente, 2003; Miller & Rollnick, 2002; Miller & Weisner, 2002). Often, the only reason they have been willing to go at all is because of external pressures of one sort or another. Furthermore, some patients do not want to participate in the staples of standard treatment—group counseling and AA—because they are not comfortable talking about their problems or otherwise simply do not like participating in groups (Cunningham, Sobell, Sobell, Agrawal, & Toneatto, 1993; Miller & Weisner, 2002; Tucker, Vuchinich, & Rippens, 2004). Quite a few individuals do not really want to adopt a goal of total abstinence or quickly lose their commitment to abstinence as a recovery goal (Appel, Ellison, Jansky, & Oldak, 2004; Humphreys & Tucker, 2002; Rapp et al., 2006; Tsogia, Copoello, & Orford, 2001). Others have had poor experiences in prior treatment episodes and, for this or other reasons, do not have much confidence in the effectiveness of standard treatment (Cunningham et al., 1993; Grant, 1997). Finally, some patients who are motivated and open to a 12-step approach simply do not have a good initial response to treatment and continue to use alcohol or drugs. These factors often lead to early dropout, which of course precludes participation in continuing care of any sort.

For those patients who do graduate from an initial level of care and are ready to make the transition to continuing care, there are relatively few options besides weekly group counseling and self-help attendance (McLellan, Carise, & Kleber, 2003). The rigidity of the treatment philosophy at this stage of recovery, the lack of any significant and viable treatment options, and limited funding for any type of continuing care lead to relatively low rates of sustained participation. It should be noted that there are people who receive continuing care for addiction problems by seeing therapists in private practice or in community mental health centers. However, there is no systematic information at this point on how many such patients there are or on their long-term outcomes. In any event, there is little in the way of mechanisms or protocols for monitoring patients with substance use disorders over extended periods of time or for "managing" their recoveries, short of isolated readmissions to acute care facilities such as emergency departments and detoxification programs.

NEW APPROACHES TO CONTINUING CARE

One of the more exciting developments in the treatment of substance use disorders over the past decade is the emergence of new adaptive models of continuing care, which take more flexible, patient-centered approaches to the management of addiction. Adaptive models of continuing care include many of the following features:

- long-term monitoring,
- more flexible protocols that can be adapted over time in response to changes in patients' symptoms and status,
- less treatment burden and greater convenience for patients,
- more attention to patient preference or choice with regard to components of care,
- use of settings other than traditional addiction specialty care programs,
- greater reliance on communication technology, and
- greater emphasis on the role of self-care in a disease management approach.

These new models have been developed with the understanding that not all individuals who might benefit from continuing care are like William in terms of their response to traditional addiction treatment. Patients such as Paul and Joan require protocols that provide considerably more flexibility in the mode of delivery, content, and timing of treatment services. Flexible protocols like this have been referred to as *adaptive treatment* in the clinical literature (Murphy, Lynch, McKay, Oslin, & Ten Have, 2007; Murphy & McKay, 2004). They are also sometimes labeled *treatment algorithms*, *dynamic treatment regimes*, or *tailored interventions*. The key characteristic of these protocols is that they can be altered, or adapted, over time, in response to changes in the patient's symptoms or functioning. When patients are doing well, the frequency and intensity of the intervention can be reduced to facilitate extended compliance. Conversely, treatment can be ratcheted up or modified in some other way when patients experience clinical deterioration. These changes are directed by carefully crafted algorithms or clinical decision trees. One of the primary goals of this book is to present and discuss recent research on these innovative approaches to the provision of continuing care in the addictions.

Outside of research studies, most clinicians do not attempt to adhere to a specified therapeutic protocol, regardless of how their patients are doing. For example, clinicians will likely attempt to modify their approach to some degree if the patient is not responding to the current intervention. However, these modifications usually do not constitute a true adaptive intervention because they do not follow from a specified set of evidence-based tailoring or monitoring variables, treatment options, and decision rules.

Although the adaptive approach to continuing care has considerable intuitive appeal to both patients and clinicians, these interventions are more complicated than traditional "fixed" approaches. Important issues and questions that quickly emerge when attempting to design an adaptive continuing care protocol include the following:

1. How is an adaptive treatment algorithm developed?
2. What kinds of therapeutic components should be included in an adaptive disease management approach?
3. When can patients be safely switched to low-intensity monitoring interventions?
4. What are the warning signs that patients may require more intensive treatment again?
5. How can compliance with adaptive interventions be increased?
6. Is there a role for patient choice or preference in the selection of treatment approaches?
7. How can clinicians evaluate the effectiveness of adaptive interventions?
8. How can evaluation be used to improve the effectiveness of adaptive interventions?
9. Do all individuals really require extended disease management?

These questions, along with potential solutions and answers, are discussed at various points in this book. Sufficient information is presented to enable a clinician or program administrator to design an adaptive intervention and to conduct research studies to support and improve the effectiveness of that intervention.

ORGANIZATION OF THIS BOOK

This book is organized into five parts: (a) the case for continuing care in addiction treatment, (b) approaches to continuing care, (c) adaptive treatment models, (d) developing and improving adaptive continuing care interventions, and (e) new developments and future directions. It also includes an appendix that presents a detailed description of an adaptive, telephone-based continuing care protocol.

Part I includes this introduction and chapter 2, which reviews evidence for patterns of repeated relapse and retreatment in treatment samples—the so-called addiction and treatment careers—and discusses the factors that influence course and outcome over time. Information from the studies reviewed in chapter 2 makes a strong case for why continuing care is necessary for many with substance use disorders.

Part II presents information on current models of continuing care. Chapter 3 provides an overview of traditional addiction treatment, with an emphasis on common approaches to continuing care, such as relapse prevention and 12-step-based group counseling. Evidence for the effectiveness of these forms of continuing care is also presented. Chapter 4 presents research on correlates of participation in continuing care and results from experimental studies that have tested interventions to increase rates of participation. Studies of the active ingredients of continuing care interventions—in other words, mediation effects—are also presented. Chapter 5 outlines a number of new approaches to extended care in the addictions that blur the distinction between initial treatment and continuing care. These models, which all provide extended care, make use of innovative strategies to sustain engagement and active participation in the interventions over time. Another notable feature of several of these care models is that they provide treatment services outside of standard specialty addiction treatment settings.

Part III is focused on adaptive treatment models. The first chapter in this part, chapter 6, describes initial attempts to individualize treatment that are based on characteristics of the patient or environment assessed at intake. This approach to tailoring treatment has been referred to as *patient-by-treatment matching*. It can been seen as a form of adaptive treatment, albeit one in which the matching is based on information collected at entrance to treatment rather than on measures of response to treatment collected at later points. Chapter 7 provides an overview of adaptive treatment models and covers key concepts and components. Some of the issues that are discussed include the difference between adaptive treatment and "matching," methods for developing adaptive treatment algorithms, the concepts of responders and nonresponders, and the use of multiple randomizations in the development of adaptive algorithms. Examples of adaptive protocols that have been developed for the treatment of other diseases and disorders, including depression, hypertension, and smoking cessation, are discussed. Adaptive treatment studies that have been conducted in the addictions over the past 10 years or so are described in chapter 8. These include studies of stepped care, extended adaptive monitoring, and adaptive continuation treatments.

Part IV includes three chapters that provide more detailed information on how to develop, evaluate, and refine adaptive continuing care interventions for clinic or practice. Chapter 9 provides an in-depth look at two adaptive approaches to the management of alcohol use disorders and one adaptive treatment for cocaine dependence, which are currently being evaluated in randomized studies. These studies are examples of two methods that can be used to develop adaptive treatment protocols: the expert consensus approach and the experimental approach. Methods and procedures used to develop the interventions in each study are described, and preliminary results are presented. In chapter 10, guidelines for selecting the key components of an adaptive protocol—the monitoring or "tailoring" variables, the menu of potential clinical interventions, and the decision rules that link tailoring variables to clinical interventions—are presented. The role of patient choice or preference in the selection of treatments is also discussed. Challenges to developing, implementing, and evaluating adaptive protocols are discussed in chapter 11. These include problems with retention and compliance, lack of viable treatment alternatives with sufficiently different mechanisms of action, timing of measurements of progress in treatment, data analytic strategies, and statistical power.

Part V addresses new developments and future directions in adaptive continuing care treatments and disease management for substance use disorders. Chapter 12 offers a look at other cutting-edge approaches to disease management in the addictions, including intensive case management of high-cost patients, recovery coaching, alternative service delivery settings, recovery models, and incorporation of new technologies. Finally, chapter 13 offers a summing up and synthesis of the main points in this book and lays out an agenda for interdisciplinary research on adaptive treatment models to further improve continuing care and disease management in the addictions.

As mentioned earlier, this book also contains an appendix that presents a detailed description of a telephone-based adaptive protocol that includes a stepped-care algorithm. Each component of the protocol is outlined, and sample scripts for therapists or counselors are provided. Additional materials for this protocol are forthcoming from Hazelden Press.

ABOUT THE TERMS USED IN THIS BOOK

As was mentioned near the beginning of this chapter, a number of terms in the addiction treatment field sometimes appear to be used interchangeably with the term *continuing care* (McKay, 2005). These include *aftercare*, *step-down care*, *stepped care*, *continuum of care*, and *disease management*. All of these terms, with the exception of *disease management*, refer to the dividing of treatment interventions into distinct phases, which differ from each other in frequency or intensity. For example, *aftercare* and *step-down care* refer to treatments of relatively brief durations that are provided after an initial, more intensive treatment phase, such as residential care or intensive outpatient treatment. *Continuing care* has also been used to denote treatment beyond the initial phase of care, but in some cases, it has implied longer term treatments. Conversely, *stepped care* and *continuum of care* refer to entire treatment protocols or systems in which patients can be moved between various intensities of care as their symptoms improve or worsen.

Although not completely synonymous with extended interventions, the term *disease management* has a similar meaning in that it implies the use of long-term interventions or at least protracted therapeutic contact of one sort or another, in the service of improved management of substance use disorders over time. Often, disease management approaches are targeted specifically to the so-called *high utilizers*—those individuals who have used a considerable amount of high-cost, acute care services, which is often an indication of poor management of a chronic disorder with standard treatment approaches.

A number of terms for substance use problems are also used in this book. *Addictive disorders* is the broadest term because it covers both abuse and dependence and refers to a number of problematic behaviors that include but are not limited to alcohol and drug use. *Alcohol and drug use disorders* and *substance use disorders* both refer to alcohol or drug use problems that reach DSM–IV diagnostic threshold for either abuse or dependence. These are the terms that are used most often in this book.

The term *abuse* refers to alcohol or drug use of sufficient severity to bring about negative consequences or the use of substances in situations in which it is hazardous to do so, such as while driving. The term *dependence* is used to indicate a more severe level of a substance use disorder, which can include features such as tolerance; withdrawal; repeated efforts to reduce substantially or quit use; giving up of important social, occupational, or recreational activities to use; and considerable time spent in activities necessary to obtain the substance, use the substance, or recover from its effects. The distinction between abuse and dependence is important because many of the treatment research studies presented in this book limited participation to individuals with alcohol or drug dependence, whereas others excluded those with dependence and instead focused on patients with abuse or heavy drinking that did not reach the level of abuse or dependence.

Finally, people in treatment for substance use disorders are referred to as *patients* rather than *clients* in this book. Both terms are used in writings about treatment for these disorders, but my unscientific take on the research literature is that the former is used more often than the latter. Therefore, to avoid confusion, I have simply used the term *patient* throughout.

FOR WHOM IS THIS BOOK?

The primary audience for this book is clinical researchers and program directors who are involved with the development and evaluation of interventions for patients with alcohol and drug use disorders. The adaptive approaches to treatment described in this book may apply as well to other chronic addictive or compulsive disorders, such as those related to gambling, food, or sex, although the necessary research has yet to be done. This book may also be of use to those who develop or evaluate interventions for other behavioral disorders, including depression, anxiety, obesity, or nicotine dependence, because much of the material on the development of adaptive interventions can apply to these disorders as well (Murphy et al., 2007; Strecher et al., 2005). Furthermore, evidence presented in chapter 7 already indicates that adaptive interventions can be effective with at least some of these disorders.

Clinicians may also find the information on the effectiveness of various continuing care interventions (see chaps. 3, 5, and 12) and strategies to increase sustained participation (see chap. 4) helpful in their work with patients who have addictive disorders. Moreover, the material describing a telephone-based adaptive continuing care protocol provided in the appendix provides a step-by-step guide on how to deliver this protocol and can also be used to supervise clinicians who are learning the protocol. Therefore, clinicians may want to focus first on the material in these chapters and in the appendix and then look at the more research-oriented sections of this book if their interests take them in that direction. To help clinicians interpret the clinical significance of research findings, indicators of the magnitude of treatment effects (i.e., small, moderate, and large) or simple percentages (i.e., 55% vs. 22% abstinent) are presented, along with statistical significance, wherever possible.

The emphasis in this book on interventions that can be modified over time in response to the changing needs of the patient may also be of interest to those providing services in various community agencies and organizations that frequently encounter and work with individuals who have substance use disorders. These include the criminal justice system, public assistance, child and youth service agencies, community medical clinics and mental health centers, employee assistance programs, and religious organizations. The "wrap-around" services provided by such agencies can be of considerable help to patients with substance use disorders, who frequently have significant problems in multiple areas that interfere with recovery. Adaptive treatment algorithms can provide a framework for integrating these additional services with addiction treatment over time.

Overall, this book emphasizes research to (a) build a strong case for the need to shift from an acute to a continuing care model of treatment, (b) document the strengths and limitations of our current approaches to continuing care, and (c) explore the potential of adaptive models of care to further improve the long-term management of substance use disorders. The focus on research is also important because current thinking on adaptive interventions posits that the best way to build an effective treatment algorithm is through the use of experimental procedures (Murphy et al., 2007). For example, the most reliable—and direct—way to determine which of two treatment options will work best for patients who do not respond to an initial intervention is to randomize the nonresponders to each option and see which one produces better outcomes with such patients.

The research procedures described in this book can also help clinicians improve the effectiveness of the adaptive continuing care protocols they develop for their clinic or practice without having to resort to randomized clinical trials. Specifically, clinicians can evaluate their protocols through the use of repeated assessments of measures of short-term outcomes, such as attendance or substance use. If the adaptive protocol does not appear to be performing as expected, the clinician or program director can institute modifications and determine whether outcomes improve with the next cohort of patients.

DOES EVERYONE NEED CONTINUING CARE?

A few additional remarks concerning the need for continuing care are in order. As mentioned earlier in this chapter, important work by Linda Sobell and colleagues demonstrated that the majority of people who recover from addictive disorders do so on their own, so to speak, or at least without the benefit of treatment or mutual help programs like AA (L. C. Sobell et al., 1993; L. C. Sobell, Ellingstad, & Sobell, 2000). A recent popular book documents many examples of the various pathways people take to recovery (Fletcher, 2001). Moreover, research has supported the effectiveness of brief interventions that may consist of as few as one or two treatment sessions (Burke, Arkowitz, & Menchola, 2003; Dunn, Deroo, & Rivara, 2001). Given these research findings, the reader may wonder whether continuing care is really needed in addiction treatment, much less long-term disease management.

It is no doubt the case that many people get over substance use disorders with little or no treatment. However, those who end up in the formal treatment system, because of either the severity of their addiction or the nature of their co-occurring problems, often cycle through periods of abstinence and abuse and end up with multiple treatment episodes over the course of their addiction careers (Hser et al., 1997, 2007). These patterns are described in more detail in chapter 2. It is not hard to make the case that more intensive and extensive forms of continuing care might be helpful for these individuals. Those who improve dramatically with minimal treatment may still benefit from low-intensity monitoring or periodic check-ups over time to help flag the onset of potential risk factors that could eventually lead to significant relapse. However, they may have little interest in standard continuing care, in which they are required to attend weekly group therapy sessions in a clinic setting. The beauty of the adaptive approach to continuing care is that it allows for differences between individuals in the nature of their recovery support needs, as well as for differences within individuals on these factors over time.

CONCLUSION

Our system that provides treatment to individuals with substance use disorders is struggling to move from an acute care orientation, characterized by relatively brief and intensive interventions that are poorly coordinated, to a continuing care-oriented model in which patients receive interventions designed to help them manage their disorders more effectively over time. Some of these continuing care interventions are effective, as is seen in chapters 3 and 5. However, it is important to note that most of the addiction treatment that is actually available in public or privately funded clinics, whether acute or continuing care, is traditional 12-step-oriented group counseling with a goal of abstinence.

Although this approach works well for some patients, at present there is little in the way of a "Plan B" for those who do not want or respond well to standard care. At this point, there is sufficient research evidence to conclude that adaptive treatment approaches have the potential to improve outcomes substantially in treatment for substance use disorders by providing evidence-based guidelines (i.e., algorithms) for modifying or adjusting treatment over time in response to changes in patient status or symptoms. Adaptive treatment may be particularly crucial for effective continuing care by (a) increasing the percentage of patients who remain in treatment long enough to receive continuing care and (b) supporting extended participation in continuing care by providing treatment that addresses current level of functioning and symptom severity while reducing patient burden whenever possible.

2

THE COURSE OF SUBSTANCE USE DISORDERS AND IMPLICATIONS FOR CONTINUING CARE

The course of substance use disorders—in other words, how they develop and wax and wane over time—and the factors that influence those processes within treatment populations have major implications for efforts to design and implement effective continuing care. For example, best practice continuing care for a disorder in which most patients recovered within 2 years might look very different from continuing care for a disorder that exhibits considerable between-individual variation in course and time to recovery. This chapter reviews and summarizes findings from studies on patterns of substance use over time, psychosocial and biological factors that confer extended vulnerability to relapse, experiences and events that appear to trigger specific relapse episodes, and positive factors that are associated with better long-term recoveries. The implications of these research findings for the long-term management of substance use disorders are discussed as well.

I am indebted to Teresa Franklin for sections she wrote on neuroscience and biological factors in relapse for an article on relapse (McKay, Franklin, Patapis, & Lynch, 2006), which have contributed to part of the Recent Developments in Neuroscience section of this chapter

Although short-term treatment outcomes are often relatively good for people who enter the formal addiction treatment system, there is still a substantial amount of problematic substance use, with rates increasing over time. For example, it is not uncommon for rates of cocaine or heroin use at post-treatment follow-ups, as indicated by self-report, urine toxicology, or hair analysis, to run as high as 40% to 60% at each follow-up (Crits-Christoph et al., 1999; McKay, Lynch, Shepard, & Pettinati, 2005; D. D. Simpson, Joe, & Broome, 2002). In addition, when outcomes are examined within individuals across multiple time periods—as opposed to group averages at one point in time—typically 25% to 50% of patients in treatment samples move back and forth between periods of abstinence and heavy substance use during follow-up (Anglin, Hser, & Grella, 1997; Dennis, Scott, & Funk, 2003; McKay & Weiss, 2001). The lack of linearity in patterns of substance use following treatment has been noted in several reports (Hufford, Witkiewitz, Shields, Kodya, & Caruso, 2003; Warren, Hawkins, & Sprott, 2003). Another indicator of chronicity is the high rate of multiple treatment experiences among patients in the treatment system. For example, in most treatment studies, at least 50% of the sample report one or more prior treatments for substance abuse, and additional episodes of treatment following relapses during follow-up are not uncommon (Dennis et al., 2003; Hser et al., 1997).

The continued vulnerability to relapse exhibited by many treatment-seeking individuals with substance use disorders appears to be a function of poor compliance with treatment and other behavioral change regimens, as well as a number of psychological, behavioral, interpersonal, and environmental risk factors (Moos, Finney, & Cronkite, 1990). There is also growing evidence that biological factors, including genetics and neurocognitive functioning, also confer extended vulnerability to relapse (Fowler, Volkow, Kassed, & Chang, 2007; Koob, 2003). At the same time, certain factors appear to offer protection against relapse. Some risk and protective factors are stable, or change relatively slowly over time. These factors raise or lower the overall risk of relapse but are not likely to determine whether a specific relapse happens at particular point in time. Factors that are the immediate precipitants of relapse have been referred to as *proximal* relapse triggers. This chapter reviews the research literature on risk and protective relapse factors and discusses the implications of these findings for continuing care interventions in the addictions.

PSYCHOSOCIAL FACTORS ASSOCIATED WITH RELAPSE AND POOR TREATMENT OUTCOME

In patients with alcohol use disorders, low readiness to change, low self-efficacy, poor coping behaviors (e.g., limited repertoire or ineffective behaviors, overreliance on avoidance coping), and greater craving have consistently been associated with poor drinking outcomes (Connors, Maisto, & Zywiak, 1996; Miller, Westerberg, Harris, & Tonigan, 1996; Moos et al., 1990; Morgenstern, Labouvie, McCrady, Kahler, & Frey, 1997; Project MATCH Research Group, 1998). It is not surprising that posttreatment scores on these measures are often much more strongly associated with subsequent drinking than pretreatment or baseline values. Poor performance while in treatment, as indicated by lack of compliance, weak therapeutic alliance, and failure to complete treatment, has also predicted worse drinking outcomes during treatment and posttreatment (Connors, Carroll, DiCelemente, Longabaugh, & Donovan, 1997; McKay et al., 2005). Lack of participation in self-help programs posttreatment has been a consistent predictor of poorer treatment outcomes (Moos & Moos, 2004; Tonigan et al., 1996; Valliant, 2003).

Moreover, greater alcohol use during follow-up has consistently been associated with, and in some cases predicted by, interpersonal problems and lack of social support for abstinence (Longabaugh, Wirtz, Beattie, Noel, & Stout, 1995; Moos et al., 1990; Weisner, Delucchi, Matzger, & Schmidt, 2003). Greater levels of life stress have also been implicated in relapse post-treatment (McKay & Weiss, 2001; Miller et al., 1996; Moos et al., 1990). For example, Moos et al. found that more problematic family environments, particularly those characterized by low cohesion, and greater life stress assessed at a 2-year follow-up were associated with worse drinking outcomes at that point and were even more strongly associated with drinking outcome 8 years later. Co-occurring psychiatric disorders, such as cocaine dependence, major depression, and antisocial personality disorder, as well as greater overall psychiatric symptom severity, have been linked to poorer drinking outcomes in some, but not all, studies (Hasin, Nunes, & Meyden 2004; McLellan, Luborsky, Woody, O'Brien, & Druley, 1983; Project MATCH Research Group, 1997).

Many of the same factors predict worse substance use outcomes in individuals with drug dependence. Studies have consistently shown that stress, craving, low motivation, low self-efficacy, lack of social support, failure to sustain participation in self-help groups and other prorecovery activities, co-occurring psychiatric disorders, and living in neighborhoods with high levels of crime and drug abuse predict worse outcomes following treatment (S. M. Hall, Havassy, & Wasserman, 1991; Havassy, Wasserman, & Hall, 1995; Hser, Grella, Hsieh, Anglin, & Brown, 1999; McKay et al., 2001; Morgenstern et al., 2003; D. D. Simpson, 2004).

Some of the psychosocial problems described here will reliably improve after individuals with substance use disorders have experienced periods of abstinence. Recovery can also bring about improvements in coping responses and self-efficacy and new socials supports that further strengthen abstinence. However, other problems—such as psychiatric disorders, interpersonal problems, lack of employment skills, and living in high-risk neighborhoods—are likely to persist or to return at later points. Data from Dennis, Foss, and Scott

(2007) demonstrated that abstinence of several years or more is necessary before improvements are observed in some areas of functioning, including employment and financial position. Good initial treatment may teach patients skills to deal with these issues, but such skills may not be retained over time or may not generalize sufficiently to address new challenges to recovery as they surface.

RECENT DEVELOPMENTS IN NEUROSCIENCE[1]

In the 1st decade of the 21st century, there have been considerable advances in our understanding of how factors such as genetics, neurochemistry, brain structure and function, and stress reactivity influence the development of addiction and propensity to relapse (Fowler et al., 2007; Goldman, Oroszi, & Ducci, 2005; Kalivas, 2007; Koob, 2006; Kreek, Nielsen, Butelman, & LaForge, 2005; Shaham & Hope, 2005). The damaging effects of alcohol and other drugs on various regions of the brain and on brain function have also been documented (Crews et al., 2005; Fowler et al., 2007). Research in these areas provides potential explanations for why some individuals have a more difficult time anticipating high-risk situations and are less likely to initiate and sustain effective coping behaviors when confronted by these situations (Kalavis, 2007; Koob, 2003; Li & Sinha, 2008). Studies have also examined the degree to which normal neurocognitive functioning is restored after periods of abstinence from alcohol or drugs.

This section of the chapter highlights some of the key findings regarding biological determinants of relapse. It should be noted that the review is selective and focuses on several factors related to brain chemistry and neurocognitive function in individuals with substance use disorders that might confer extended vulnerability to relapse. The degree to which neurocognitive functioning improves with extended abstinence is also addressed.

Biological Factors in Addiction and Relapse Vulnerability

Animal and human studies have suggested that problems in the prefrontal cortical area of the brain, and regions functionally and anatomically connected to it, are key factors in vulnerability to addiction and likely implicated in relapse as well (Fowler et al., 2007; Franklin et al., 2002; Kalivas, 2007; Koob, 2006). These regions, which include the anterior cingulated cortex and the orbitofrontal cortex, are located in the front of the brain and contribute to what is referred to as *executive function* (Nestler, 2005). That is,

[1]Portions of this section are adapted from "Conceptual, Methodological, and Analytical Issues in the Study of Relapse," by J. R. McKay, T. R. Franklin, N. Patapis, and K. G. Lynch, 2006, *Clinical Psychology Review*, 26, pp. 116–118. Copyright 2006 by Elsevier. Adapted with permission.

these regions are involved in planning and exert inhibitory control over other parts of the brain, thereby reducing impulsivity. It is not entirely clear whether the poor performance of the prefrontal cortex precedes addiction or is the result of it, but difficulty in inhibiting urges, including craving to use drugs, no doubt plays a role in relapse (Li & Sinha, 2008).

Chronic use of substances such as cocaine also leads to changes in reward learning processes (Kalivas, 2007). Increases in the neurotransmitter dopamine play a key role in the rewarding properties of cocaine and other drugs of abuse (i.e., euphoria), as well as in more naturally occurring rewards (Fowler et al., 2007; Koob, 2006; Nestler, 2005). Cocaine use produces increases in dopamine that are far greater in size and duration than those produced by naturally occurring rewarding stimuli such as food, sex, or social cooperation. Moreover, exposure to cocaine continues to produce these huge increases in dopamine, whereas exposure to naturally occurring rewards tends to lead to smaller and smaller releases of dopamine, unless the reward changes in some way to make it once again novel (Kalivas, 2007). Therefore, over time drug use results in a pathological form of reward seeking, in which the addict continues to find drug use highly rewarding but gets less and less enjoyment out of anything else (Kalivas, 2007; Koob, 2006; Li & Sinha, 2008).

The relatively high rewarding properties of substances of abuse over more natural reinforcers may also explain the tendency of alcohol or drug abusers to focus attention on stimuli related to substance use to a greater degree than someone who does not abuse substances. This process has been referred to as *attentional bias* (Waters, Shiffman, Bradley, & Mogg, 2003). Moreover, there is even evidence that the limbic regions of the brain respond to presentations of drug cues that are so brief (e.g., 33 ms) that the individual with a substance use disorder is not consciously aware of having seen them (Childress et al., 2008). After addiction has been established, changes in the brain lead to the increased salience of drugs and cues associated with them and to relatively stronger positive reactions to drugs compared with naturally occurring rewards. These changes are not likely to be quickly reversed during periods of abstinence.

Increased biological reactivity to stress appears to be another important factor in the maintenance of addiction and in relapse (Koob, 2006; Li & Sinha, 2008; Nestler, 2005). Initial studies with cocaine-dependent individuals indicated that exposure to stress and drug cues each resulted in significant increases in cocaine craving and in the stress hormones adrenocorticotropic hormone and cortisol (Sinha, Catapano, & O'Malley, 1999; Sinha et al., 2003). Moreover, acute cortisol administration triggered craving in cocaine abusers (Elman, Lukas, Karlsgodt, Gasic, & Breiter, 2003). Koob (2000) also proposed that heightened corticotropin-releasing factor response in alcoholics during protracted abstinence may be a factor in increased risk for relapse over time.

In contrast, a recent study found that reduced reactivity to stress, as indicated by lower cortisol levels after a laboratory stress inducing paradigm, predicted a greater likelihood of early relapse in alcoholic males (Junghanns et al., 2003). This finding is in keeping with research in children, which has shown that reduced basal cortisol concentrations have been associated with aggressivity (Tennes, Kreye, Avitable, & Wells, 1986), hostility (Tennes & Kreye, 1985), and conduct disorder severity (Vanyukov et al., 1993). Moreover, lower cortisol levels in children have been shown to be associated with higher conduct disorder symptom counts and higher antisocial personality symptom counts in their fathers (Vanyukov et al., 1993). It is therefore possible that dysregulation of the hypothalamic–pituitary–adrenal (HPA) axis in the stress-response system, as indicated by either reduced or increased stress reactivity, could play a role in relapse. These apparently contradictory findings may also reflect differences in the effects of chronic versus acute stress.

Increasing evidence suggests a genetic basis for some of the abnormalities in neurocognitive function that are associated with addiction. First, it is clear that genes contribute to vulnerability to substance use disorders, with estimates of heritability ranging from 30% to 72% (Goldman et al., 2005; Kreek et al., 2005). One can surmise that many of the genes that contribute to increased vulnerability to become addicted in the first place may also play a role in extended vulnerability to subsequent relapse following periods of abstinence. For example, genes that influence personality dimensions such as impulsivity, risk taking, and novelty seeking may contribute to both higher rates of addiction and greater vulnerability to relapse (Kreek et al., 2005). Genetic factors also appear to influence the ways in which various drugs of abuse affect physiology and subjective reactions, such as craving and degree of euphoria (Franklin et al., 2008; Oslin et al., 2003), which could contribute to extended vulnerability to relapse. Finally, genetic factors appear to influence how reactive the stress-response system is, through alterations in the HPA axis (Kreek et al., 2005). Obviously, genetically based vulnerabilities that increase the risk of relapse persist for extended periods—if not throughout the life span.

Is Recovery of Normal Neurocognitive Processes Possible?

It is clear at this point that heavy use of alcohol and other drugs can damage structures in the brain and interfere with optimal neurofunctioning (Crews et al., 2005; Fowler et al., 2007). Researchers have begun to study the degree to which deficits in brain structure and function associated with substance use normalize following periods of abstinence, which has major implications for treatment issues, such as the focus and duration of continuing care. For example, methamphetamine has been found to be neurotoxic to dopamine terminals when administered to laboratory animals. Volkow et al. (2001) studied the effect of extended abstinence in five methamphetamine users on dopamine transporters in one brain region, the striatum, using positron emission tomography (PET) scans. Brain dopamine transporters were evaluated during short abstinence (< 6 months) and then retested during protracted abstinence (12–17 months). The results of the testing showed significant increases with protracted abstinence. However, neuropsychological tests did not improve to the same extent, which suggests that the increase of the DA transporters was not sufficient for complete recovery of function. These findings have treatment implications because they suggest that protracted abstinence may reverse some—but not all—of methamphetamine-induced alterations in brain DA terminals.

In a follow-up study, again with methamphetamine users, Wang et al. (2004) found evidence of partial recovery after protracted abstinence of thalamic metabolism but not striatal metabolism. The increase in thalamic metabolism was associated with improved performance in motor and verbal memory tests. These researchers speculated that the persistent decreases in striatal metabolism in methamphetamine abusers could reflect long-lasting changes in dopamine cell activity and could account for the persistence of problems with motivation and affect in detoxified methamphetamine abusers. The recovery of thalamic metabolism could reflect adaptation responses to compensate for the dopamine deficits, and the associated improvement in neuropsychological performance further indicates its functional significance. Taken together, the results of these two studies suggest that although protracted abstinence may reverse some of the methamphetamine-induced alterations in brain function, other deficits persist (Wang et al., 2004).

There is now convincing evidence in studies of humans and animals that binge drinking leads to damage to parts of the brain that are involved with executive functioning, visuospatial abilities, and postural stability (Crews et al., 2005; Monti et al., 2005). Heavy drinking appears to be particularly damaging to the brains of adolescents (Crews, Braun, Hoplight, Switzer, & Knapp, 2000). Fortunately, recovery from alcoholism is associated with a partial reversal of some of these deficits (Crews et al., 2005; Fowler et al., 2007). However, further relapses may limit these improvements (Pfefferbaum et al., 1995), and some deficits may persist even during more extended periods of abstinence.

Intriguing research by Obernier, White, Swartzwelder, and Crews (2002) used an animal model to study the effects of binge drinking. Rats consumed alcohol at binge levels over a 4-day period and were then "abstinent" for several days. In subsequent behavioral testing, the animals were able to learn new tasks as well as rats that had not been binging, but they were not as able to change their approach when the requirements of the task changed. Instead, they perseverated in their old, now ineffective, behavior. If these sorts of difficulties with executive function in the brain persist, it could at least partially explain the apparent difficulty some alcoholics have in changing their approach to dealing with risky situations when a particular coping response is no longer effective.

In summary, the research performed to date strongly suggests that relapse to substances of abuse is related to a number of neurocognitive factors, including irregularities in the reward system, poor inhibitory control linked to problems in the prefrontal cortex and related regions of the brain, and abnormal reactivity to stress. These factors appear to be genetically determined, are a result of chronic alcohol or drug use, or are a combination of both. Some of these deficits appear to improve with periods of abstinence, but others do not, suggesting long-term increased vulnerability to relapse. If deficits do indeed persist over prolonged periods of time, even after abstinence is achieved, extended interventions that continue to address issues such as impulsivity and reduced ability to learn from prior behavior may be necessary.

ASSESSMENT AND ANALYSIS OF IMMEDIATE ANTECEDENTS OF RELAPSE[2]

The literature reviewed so far in this chapter has focused on relatively stable factors, such as coping skills, interpersonal relations, ability to control impulses, and so forth, that are associated with risk for relapse or that predict the likelihood of relapse at some later point. However, these models do not really address the question of why someone relapses at a specific point in time. The influential cognitive–behavioral model of relapse (Brownell, Marlatt, Lichtenstein, & Wilson, 1986; Marlatt & Gordon, 1985; Witkiewitz & Marlatt, 2004) attempts to provide a microanalysis of the relapse process. The model postulates that one of two processes occurs when a substance abuser encounters a high-risk situation, such as negative mood, interpersonal problems, invitations to drink or use drugs, and so forth. If the individual has high self-efficacy, or the belief that he or she can manage that particular situation without using alcohol or drugs (i.e., relapsing), a coping response is performed, and relapse is avoided. However, if the individual has lower self-efficacy, a coping response is not performed and relapse ensues. Therefore, in this model relapse is seen largely as a function of whether one (a) encounters high-risk situations and (b) is able to mount an effective coping response. Other cognitive features of the model include outcome expectancies (i.e., what will happen as a result of either substance use or the exercise of a coping behavior) and attributions for one's behavior (McKay et al., 2006).

Since the mid 1990s, the cognitive–behavioral model of relapse has been broadened to include some of the factors discussed earlier in this chapter, including enduring personal characteristics, background variables, and

---

[2]Portions of this section are adapted from "Conceptual, Methodological, and Analytical Issues in the Study of Relapse," by J. R. McKay, T. R. Franklin, N. Patapis, and K. G. Lynch, 2006, *Clinical Psychology Review*, 26, pp. 110, 113–116. Copyright 2006 by Elsevier. Adapted with permission.

life stress (Donovan, 1996; Miller et al., 1996; Sinha, 2001). The more recent work described briefly here has also emphasized biological factors that may moderate risk of relapse, including genetics, poor executive functioning, and heightened stress reactivity. These findings are not incompatible with the cognitive–behavioral model of relapse; rather, they can be seen as complementing it. For example, the ability of some individuals to mount a successful coping behavior in a high-risk situation might be diminished by particularly strong craving or poor impulse control, both of which could be mediated by biological factors (McKay et al., 2006). Moreover, recent stressful life events could also reduce one's ability to cope effectively in high-risk situations (Sinha, 2001).

One of the limitations of the cognitive–behavioral model of relapse is that it has not been possible to test it adequately using conventional questionnaires and interviews. Because substance abusers are usually not available for interview immediately before or during relapses, data on the precipitants of the episodes has usually been gathered through retrospective interviews, often administered weeks or months after the relapse episode. Such data are likely to be biased or incomplete (Hammersley, 1994; McKay, 1999; Shiffman et al., 1997).

To get around the limitations of retrospective interviews and obtain more accurate and complete data on the experience of individuals immediately before and even during relapses, Shiffman and Stone (1998) developed a method referred to as *ecological momentary assessment* (EMA). This approach makes use of small, handheld computers, often referred to as *electronic diaries*, to obtain data on substance use, internal states, situational factors, and other aspects of experience before, during, and after lapses and relapses. With regard to the study of relapse to addictive behavior, EMA has been used primarily with smokers. The primary advantage of this approach is the tremendous flexibility in data collection that can be written into the software of the units. For example, participants can be signaled on a random basis to enter data on their current internal states, experiences, and coping behaviors. Moreover, they can enter data while experiencing strong urges to smoke or use substances, as well as after they have started to use. These data make it possible to examine factors in the days or even hours before relapse episodes that differentiate these periods from episodes of temptation that did not result in relapse and from periods of stable continued abstinence. Moreover, the data can provide information on factors associated with the duration of lapses and whether they turn into full-blown relapses.

The initial EMA studies of smoking relapses were done by Shiffman and colleagues in the middle 1990s. These studies showed that smoking lapses were associated with increased urges and negative affect, environments conducive to smoking, and the failure to perform some sort of coping response (Shiffman, Paty, Gnys, Kassel, & Hickcox, 1996). Furthermore, this earlier research demonstrated that the progression from first smoking lapse to full relapse was influenced by factors such as urge to "give up" attempts to not smoke, degree to which the lapse was precipitated by stress, and coping efforts (Shiffman, Hickcox, et al., 1996).

A study on smoking relapse by Shiffman and Waters (2004) illustrates the power of this methodology. Data on daily stress (i.e., negative and positive events) and negative affect were obtained from electronic diaries. Results indicated that day-to-day changes in stress and negative affect did not predict smoking lapses the next day, even when the participant later attributed the lapse to stress or negative affect. However, data collected through electronic diaries indicated that there were significant increases in negative affect in the hours before smoking lapses occurred. This finding strongly suggests that to understand the determinants of a particular relapse, it is necessary to obtain accurate data on internal states and experiences very close in time to the onset of the episode.

Another study by Shiffman et al. (2000) explored the role of self-efficacy in smoking relapses. In this study, self-efficacy was assessed a week before the targeted quit date using a questionnaire, and then repeatedly through electronic diaries over the 4 weeks following smoking cessation. The results indicated that self-efficacy remained high before the first smoking lapse and decreased after that. Although daily self-efficacy did predict the likelihood of a lapse the next day, this relationship was actually accounted for by individual differences in self-efficacy assessed at baseline through the questionnaire. However, daily self-efficacy, assessed with electronic diaries, did predict the likelihood that lapses would progress to full relapses. It should be noted that this study obtained both distal (i.e., before quit date) and proximal (i.e., daily) measures of self-efficacy. The results suggest that distal measures of self-efficacy are a good indication of the likelihood of substance use at some point in the future, whereas proximal measures of self-efficacy predict how severe the next episode of use will be.

POSITIVE FACTORS IN LONG-TERM RECOVERY

Studies have also examined the correlates of good long-term recoveries, with a focus on positive factors. Longitudinal studies by Vaillant and colleagues suggest that long-term recovery is associated with several factors, including substitute dependencies (e.g., meditation, compulsive hobbies), new social supports, and increased hope and self-esteem (Vaillant, 1998, 2003; Vaillant et al., 1983). According to Vaillant (1998, 2003), participation in religion and self-help programs can be particularly useful for rekindling hope and rebuilding self-esteem.

Moos and Moos (2007) reported on findings from a 16-year longitudinal study of 461 individuals who sought help for alcohol problems. Several factors were predictive of better outcomes over the follow-up period. People who got treatment in a timely fashion had better outcomes over the 16 years than those who either delayed entry into treatment or remained untreated. Participants who participated in self-help for at least 27 weeks in the 1st year had significantly higher rates of remission at Year 16 (70%) than those who did not attend Alcoholics Anonymous (AA) in the 1st year (43%) or those who attended between 1 and 26 weeks (57%). Other factors assessed at 3- and 8-year follow-ups that predicted higher remission rates in subsequent follow-ups were higher self-efficacy, approach coping, and support from friends. Recovery-oriented social networks and self-help participation also predicted decreased alcohol use over a 5-year period in samples of dependent and problem drinkers in a study by Weisner, Delucchi, Matzger, and Schmidt (2003). However, virtually all studies with longer follow-ups find that participation in AA and other mutual-help organizations decreases over time.

Qualitative data from two of our continuing care studies at the University of Pennsylvania (McKay et al., 1999; McKay, Lynch, Shepard, & Pettinati, 2005) are in agreement with the results of Vaillant's work. Our research staff conducted extensive semistructured interviews with some of the participants from these studies who reported total abstinence over the 2-year follow-up and for whom corroborating evidence of abstinence was also available (e.g., from urine toxicology screens and collateral informants). This sample consisted of 10 men and 3 women. Of these individuals, 10 were dependent on cocaine and alcohol when they came into treatment, 1 on cocaine only, and 2 on alcohol only.

In response to the question "What two things do you believe have been most important in helping you stay sober?" the most common responses were a higher power (77%) and attending self-help meetings (54%). Various other aspects of self-help programs were also reported, including working the steps, having a sponsor, prayer, and adhering to the "one day at a time" philosophy. Other factors reported were family, living in a recovery house, "really wanting it," treatment, avoidance of high-risk situations, and fear.

Participants were also asked about what their typical day was like. The majority of participants reported that most of their days were spent working; some, in fact, had two jobs. Going to self-help meetings was also frequently reported, as were other activities, including hobbies and seeing family. Participants reported a smattering of other things, including prayer, church, meditation, housework, volunteer work, exercise, and education. With regard to leisure time and recreational activities, they reported going to movies, spending time with friends and family, attending self-help functions, watching TV, playing sports, reading, playing games, taking trips, going out to eat, and walking.

It is notable that this balance of work and various other activities seems fairly typical of individuals who are functional members of society and is in stark contrast to the lives these patients were living when they were using alcohol and drugs. As one of our participants put it, "I bowl. Once in awhile

I go to the movies . . . normal stuff . . . out to dinner. I didn't do any of that stuff when I was drinking. I mean zero." Similar findings were obtained in a British alcohol treatment study in which participants attributed their recoveries to a combination of seeing the benefits of a new alcohol-free lifestyle, throwing themselves into other activities, taking advantage of social supports, and changing their cognitions regarding alcohol use, in part through using tools they had obtained in treatment (Orford et al., 2006).

SUMMARY OF RESEARCH FINDINGS ON RISK AND PROTECTIVE FACTORS

Individuals with a history of substance use disorders who have entered the formal treatment system often struggle with a number of factors that place them at heightened risk of relapse, in some cases for considerable lengths of time. Some of these factors are relatively slow to change, such as interpersonal problems, co-occurring psychiatric disorders, employment problems, living in impoverished neighborhoods, poor executive functioning, attentional biases, heightened stress response, and other neurocognitive problems. Moreover, risk factors based on genetics are unlikely to change at all. However, some relapse vulnerability factors are quite dynamic and can change relatively rapidly—over periods as short as a few hours or as long as several days or weeks. These factors include mood, stress, craving, motivation, and self-efficacy.

Most positive factors associated with recovery are relatively slow to change and require ongoing effort and support to prevent deterioration. These include the development of social networks that support recovery, substitute dependencies and passions, improved coping responses, and employment and other activities that provide a sense of worth, meaning, and self-esteem.

IMPLICATIONS FOR THE DEVELOPMENT OF EFFECTIVE CONTINUING CARE MODELS

The research findings reviewed in this chapter on the course of substance use disorders and the factors that appear to influence these trajectories suggest the following conclusions:

1. Patients who enter the formal treatment system tend to have relapse vulnerabilities that persist or are likely to reappear, such as neurocognitive deficits, co-occurring problems, skills deficits, poor coping behaviors, employment problems, inconsistent motivation, and environmental risk factors. Treatment generally cannot eliminate all these risk factors but may help patients to manage them when they are present.

2. Clinically significant changes in some relapse vulnerabilities (e.g., mood) can occur rapidly, over periods of several hours.
3. Positive, or prerecovery, behaviors are important for long-term recovery but tend to drop off over time. Many people may need extended monitoring, support, and positive reinforcement to help them sustain such behaviors.

These findings may explain why initial and continuing care treatments derived from an acute care model are of limited effectiveness in the long-term management of drug dependence. Specifically, vulnerability to relapse remains relatively high for significant periods of time after standard treatment protocols of 3 to 6 months have ended (Dennis et al., 2003; McLellan et al., 2000). Better management requires longer periods of continued contact with the patient (Dennis & Scott, 2007; McLellan, McKay, Forman, Cacciola, & Kemp, 2005; Wagner et al., 2001) to address flagging motivation, increased craving, poor compliance with lifestyle changes and self- and mutual-help participation, limitations in neurocognitive function, continued biological vulnerability to stress and other factors, and various other problems that arise. Of course, extended contact must not impose undue burden on patients or poor compliance will result, and it must be relatively economical.

These findings also suggest that in the case of each person with a substance use disorder, there are likely to be shifts in risk and protective factors over time. Some of these shifts will occur slowly, over months or even years, whereas others may occur quite rapidly, over days or even hours. Some shifts will be sufficiently major to require changes in level of care—for example, an individual who sporadically attended AA meetings while experiencing a prolonged relapse may require intensive outpatient or residential care to return to abstinence. Other shifts in risk or protective factors, however, may be addressed successfully by altering the types of interventions being delivered within the same level of care. For example, decreases in motivation for abstinence could be addressed by greater use of motivational interviewing techniques, and skills deficits or cognitive biases that are associated with repeated relapse episodes might be modified through cognitive–behavioral therapy.

Finally, poor treatment compliance and outcomes can also reflect the patient's lack of interest in or preference for that particular kind of treatment. A common example of this is the patient who attends AA faithfully for a few months but then decides it is not for him anymore. The diligent counselor can continue to urge the patient to go to AA, but at some point it makes sense to have a "Plan B" to recommend to the patient. Continued pressure on the patient to do what he does not want to do is likely to result in further compliance problems and possibly bad outcomes.

The fact that some risk and protective factors as well as patient preferences are likely to change over time during the course of recovery, whereas others persist for long periods, strongly suggests that continuing care protocols need to be highly flexible and patient-centered. Continuing care based on these principles is more likely to promote extended compliance and good outcomes than are interventions that are relatively rigid in structure. The three chapters in Part II present findings from research on the effectiveness of standard continuing care models, mechanisms of change in continuing care and methods to increase participation, and extended models of care that blur the distinction between initial treatment and continuing care. In these research findings, readers will see initial evidence that treatments that more directly address the specific challenges inherent in managing chronic disorders do in fact generate better substance use outcomes than other interventions.

II

APPROACHES TO
CONTINUING CARE

3

TRADITIONAL APPROACHES TO ADDICTION TREATMENT AND CONTINUING CARE

Continuing care was originally conceived of as a lower intensity treatment phase that followed a more intensive, first phase of care. Back in the 1970s and 1980s, continuing care generally followed episodes of inpatient or residential treatment and was often located in a separate facility. However, by the late 1990s, day hospitals and intensive outpatient programs (IOPs) were increasingly used as an initial level of care replacing residential treatment (McLellan & Meyers, 2004). At that point, individuals with substance use disorders typically had to have severe co-occurring psychiatric or medical problems to be eligible for residential treatment, unless they had excellent health insurance or the resources to self-pay. Therefore, in the outpatient addiction treatment model, continuing care was often provided at the same facility as the initial level of care and generally represented an extension of

Portions of this chapter have been adapted from "Continuing Care Research: What We Have Learned and Where We Are Going," by J. R. McKay, 2009, *Journal of Substance Abuse Treatment, 36*, pp. 132–137. Copyright 2009 by Elsevier. Adapted with permission.

the treatment provided in the first phase, albeit at a lower frequency and intensity.

This chapter describes the types of continuing care interventions that have typically been available to patients following the completion of initial forms of treatment: self- and mutual-help meetings and standard addiction group counseling. Several individual or conjoint continuing care treatment approaches are also described, including cognitive–behavioral therapy (CBT), 12-step facilitation (TSF), and couples or family therapy. Research findings regarding the effectiveness of continuing care interventions are also presented, with a focus on 20 controlled studies published since the late 1980s. All of these studies followed the traditional continuing care model, in which patients first complete an initial, more intensive, phase of care before becoming eligible for continuing care. Finally, several conclusions are drawn regarding the characteristics of effective continuing care interventions.

RESIDENTIAL TREATMENT AND AFTERCARE

The classic approach to addiction treatment is the Alcoholics Anonymous (AA)–12-step-oriented 28-day rehabilitation program, followed by referral to AA for continuing care. This approach, which is often referred to as the *Minnesota model*, was developed at Hazelden and other residential programs and became popular in the 1960s (Anderson, McGovern, & Dupont, 1999; McElrath, 1997). The Minnesota model approach was progressive in some ways, in that it conceptualized addiction as a disease rather than a bad habit or a free choice, recognized that extended vulnerability to relapse was the norm, and argued for the importance of long-term treatment—although this treatment was provided outside the health care system, through self-help (White, 1998).

However, the Minnesota model took a "one size fits all" approach to treating addiction, making little attempt to individualize treatment to particular patients' characteristics or needs. Moreover, the AA approach that was the foundation for the Minnesota model divided alcoholics up into two main groups. One group consisted of those individuals who were "ready" to change and willing to follow the recommendations of the AA program, usually after having tried every other possible approach without success. AA practically guaranteed abstinence to these people—"If you work the program, it will work for you!" The second group included those alcoholics who were not willing to embrace the AA philosophy and rules for living. For them, there really was no other viable treatment option.

Unfortunately, this produced an "our way or the highway" mentality in addiction treatment, which was antithetical to the idea of individualized treatment. There was only one road to recovery, and counselors were taught to confront and hound patients until they saw the light. It should be noted that the Minnesota model is much more flexible at this point, especially with regard to continuing care issues. However, the approach is still problematic for those patients who are not willing to adopt AA.

Given the relapsing nature of the disorder, individuals receiving treatment for substance abuse were generally urged to participate in some form of continuing care after their initial phase of treatment had ended. When most substance abuse treatment was delivered in inpatient or residential settings, continuing care usually consisted of outpatient aftercare group therapy sessions and participation in self- or mutual-help programs such as AA. Aftercare was intended to ease the transition from the controlled therapeutic environment, particularly for people who traveled to another locale to attend a 28-day rehabilitation program and to maintain progress achieved in the inpatient or residential program. These aftercare groups were generally extensions of the treatment patients had received in the residential programs in that they stressed the AA approach to recovery and provided continued support for participation in self- or mutual-help programs.

SHIFT TO OUTPATIENT TREATMENT

By the 1990s, more and more addiction treatment was provided in outpatient settings. The vast majority of these programs followed the approach of the Minnesota model: The treatment content was based on the 12-step approach and delivered through group therapy, and didactic material was provided through videos and lectures. However, the treatment was lengthened beyond 30 days and often segmented into intensive versus standard outpatient treatment. Continuing care became the standard outpatient treatment that was offered to patients who completed the initial phase of more intensive outpatient treatment. Other approaches to addiction treatment, such as CBT, motivational interviewing, behavioral couples therapy, and contingency management, were developed, although their use has been restricted primarily to research studies. Some of these interventions have also been used as continuing care, or elements of them have been included in more standard continuing care interventions (e.g., relapse prevention).

Currently, most substance abuse treatment is provided in outpatient settings (McLellan, Carise, & Kleber, 2003; McLellan & Meyers, 2004; Substance Abuse and Mental Health Services Administration [SAMHSA], 2002, 2008), with residential or inpatient treatment restricted to those with severe co-occurring medical or psychiatric problems (American Society of Addiction Medicine, 2001). In the outpatient model, patients participate in an initial treatment phase with a planned duration of 30 to 60 days, which typically ranges from two (i.e., standard outpatient) or three (i.e., intensive outpatient) contacts per week up to daily contact (i.e., day hospital; SAMHSA, 2008). Patients who complete this phase then enter standard outpatient treatment, which usually consists of one contact per week. Continuing care treatment in the outpatient model is usually delivered through group sessions, focused on substance use and oriented around the 12 steps of mutual- and self-help programs.

One of the major differences between the older residential care model and contemporary outpatient rehabilitation is that significant percentages of patients continue to use drugs or drink during IOP. For example, in one of our continuing care studies, approximately 20% of the patients who completed IOP and entered the study had failed to achieve remission from current cocaine dependence during IOP (McKay et al., 1997). Studies have consistently indicated that patients who fail to achieve at least several consecutive weeks of abstinence early in treatment have significantly poorer longer term substance use outcomes than those who do achieve early abstinence (Carroll et al., 1994; Higgins, Badger, & Budney, 2000; McKay et al., 1999). Therefore, continuing care programs in contemporary, outpatient-based service delivery systems are asked to manage a wide variety of patients, ranging from those who have already achieved abstinence outside of a controlled environment to those who have not yet achieved any meaningful abstinence at all.

CONTINUING CARE INTERVENTIONS

Most of the continuing care available to patients with substance use disorders has been provided in self-help meetings or in group counseling sessions, which are described in this section. Also described are two individual approaches, CBT and TSF, and one conjoint approach, behavioral couples therapy (BCT). These three interventions are not as widely available but have been evaluated in many research studies.

Self-Help Programs

The most available self-help programs for those with substance use disorders are AA, Narcotics Anonymous (NA), and Cocaine Anonymous (CA). These programs are all peer led and abstinence oriented, and they can provide considerable social support for recovery (Humphreys, 2004; White & Kurtz, 2006). Active participation in AA and related programs involves frequent attendance at meetings, regular out-of-meeting contacts with others in the program, and a commitment to the 12-step program of recovery. The 12 steps provide a spiritual and behavioral guide to self-improvement and recovery. Some of the steps require daily effort, such as admitting powerlessness over alcohol and other drugs (Step 1) and turning one's will over to a higher power (Step 3). Conversely, other steps are completed and then not repeated for some period of time, such as making a searching and fearless moral inventory (Step 4), describing the inventory to another person (Step 5), and making amends for past bad behavior (Step 9).

There are several types of meetings (Forman, 2002), and participants are advised to go to all types. Speaker meetings are often relatively large meetings in which one to three invited speakers tell their own personal story of descent into addiction and eventual recovery through the 12-step program. At speaker meetings, the other participants listen and typically say little. At discussion meetings, the group leader selects a topic and makes a few opening comments, and then each participant in turn is given an opportunity to offer comments on the topic or talk about anything else that is on his or her mind. A variant of discussion meetings is the 12-step meeting in which the topic each week is one of the 12 steps. Meetings are held in a variety of places, including churches, hospitals, members' houses, and clubhouses. In large cities, it is usually possible to find meetings within a short distance of practically any location at all hours of the day and evening.

Twelve-step self-help meetings vary considerably in the makeup of regular attendees. Meetings in business centers of cities and in affluent suburbs are attended largely by professionals who are in recovery. There are traditional meetings, attended for the most part by older alcoholics who do not have co-occurring drug problems. There are also meetings for other types of substance abusers, including young people, women, nonsmokers, and individuals with co-occurring psychiatric disorders. Individual meetings can be quite different with regard to attendees' attitudes toward psychiatric medication and tolerance for discussions about matters other than drinking and drug use. New members of self-help programs are often told to try other meetings if they feel out of place at the ones they first attend (Forman, 2002).

Individuals who are active in 12-step-oriented self-help programs attribute their effectiveness to various components of the programs (Humphreys, 2004; White & Kurtz, 2006). For example, some people stress the spiritual aspects, including admitting powerlessness over alcohol and drugs, turning to God or another higher power and to prayer to lift the compulsion to drink or use drugs. Conversely, others point to the tremendous social support provided by regular attendance at meetings and out-of-meeting contact with others in the program. Still others focus on the aspects of the 12-step program that rehabilitate character and reduce self-involvement, such as making amends, helping others recover, and engaging in daily efforts toward greater humility and acceptance and less grandiosity.

The vast majority of addiction treatment programs follow the 12 steps of AA (McLellan et al., 2003). While in treatment, patients are typically expected to attend three or more meetings per week and to begin to "work" the 12-step program. This often means making some progress toward the first four steps, selecting an initial sponsor who will serve as a mentor and connection to self-help meetings and others in the program, and developing a list of meetings to attend regularly once treatment has ended. Unfortunately, many patients are initially resistant to self-help participation, and a high percentage of those who attend meetings at first stop going relatively quickly. Reported reasons for not participating in AA and related programs include their focus on spirituality, the requirement of a commitment to total abstinence, and the use of a group format. Some individuals also report difficulty relating to other members or having the sense that they do not belong. Other self-help programs are available to those who object to various aspects of 12-step-oriented programs. These include Rational Recovery, Self-Management and Recovery Training, SOS/LifeRing Secular Recovery, and Women for Sobriety (Humphreys, 2004).

The results of a number of reviews suggest that individuals who regularly attend self-help programs and participate in a full range of related program activities, such as talking with a sponsor, getting together with other program members outside of meetings, and being a sponsor, have better alcohol and drug use outcomes than those with little or no self-help participation (Kissin, McLeod, & McKay, 2003; Moos & Moos, 2007; Tonigan et al., 1996). However, these effects could simply reflect self-selection, with more motivated and successful patients also attending more self-help. Unfortunately, there are few randomized studies of self-help programs, in part because of concerns about the ethics of assigning some study participants to a no-AA control condition. An excellent review of various self-help programs and evidence concerning their effectiveness is found in Humphreys (2004).

12-Step-Oriented Group Counseling

The most common form of continuing care, outside of self-help meetings, is group counseling with a 12-step focus or orientation. These groups are offered in a many addiction specialty treatment programs and mental health centers, usually in the form of one or two 60- to 90-minute sessions per week (Crits-Christoph et al., 1999). The groups usually have one leader, although coleaders are not unusual, particularly when the clinic has trainees. Although these groups are not standardized and typically are not guided by a manual, they do tend to have a number of common elements. These include reports by patients of their current status, including any recent alcohol or drug use; feedback, support, and sometimes confrontation from other group members and counselors; attention to progress in working on specific steps in the 12-step program and attendance at 12-step meetings; and planning of leisure activities during the week and especially on the weekend, along with general structuring of time in ways that promote recovery.

These groups usually feature rolling admissions, so that they always contain a mix of new and more experienced patients. The size of the groups can vary considerably, although most clinics strive for around 10 to 15 patients per group. The planned duration of these continuing care groups is usually in the range of 3 to 6 months, although longer stays are possible in some settings. However, dropout rates are fairly high, with most studies indicating that approximately 50% of patients stop attending before 3 months (McKay et al., 1999; McKay, Lynch, et al., 2004).

One aspect of this form of continuing care that can be somewhat confusing is that the same basic format—one or two groups per week—can also be used as a primary treatment for lower severity patients and those who do not want more intensive treatments such as IOP or residential care. In that context, it is usually referred to as *standard outpatient care* (OP as opposed to IOP). Therefore, in some clinics the patients who are attending these groups are a mix of graduates of IOPs and patients who have entered the system at the OP level.

Individual Therapies

Some continuing care is provided through individual counseling and psychotherapy. For example, many mental health professionals in solo or group private practices (e.g., social workers, psychologists, psychiatrists) have at least a few individuals in their caseloads who are in recovery from addiction. For such patients, their therapy sessions could certainly be considered a form of continuing care. However, there is virtually no systematic information on how many patients in recovery from addiction are being seen in private practices.

Individual counseling or therapy is not often offered in specialty clinics because patients have poor or nonexistent insurance coverage and cannot afford large out-of-pocket expenses. However, several individual continuing care therapies have been developed for research studies. These include CBT and TSF.

Cognitive–Behavioral Therapy

The principal goals of CBT for addictive disorders are to identify and address biased and maladaptive beliefs and attitudes that contribute to the development and maintenance of addiction and to improve cognitive and behavioral coping responses to high-risk situations (Carroll, 1998; Monti, Abrams, Kadden, & Cooney, 1999). The purported mechanisms of action, or mediators, in CBT include self-efficacy (Bandura, 1991) and behavioral skills. Specifically, correcting biases and maladaptive beliefs and improving coping skills are hypothesized to increase self-efficacy. This leads to successful coping in high-risk situations, which in turn further raises self-efficacy.

CBT often begins with a functional analysis, which is a fine-grained examination of the factors leading up to a recent episode of substance use. The goal of the functional analysis is to determine the specific situations in which an individual has been prone to use substances. For example, one person may use when depressed, whereas another may be more likely to use after interpersonal difficulties. After determining when the patient is most likely to use, the treatment moves on to help the patient learn to recognize and anticipate high-risk situations and to learn better means of coping with them. A version of CBT that has been used primarily as continuing care is relapse prevention (RP; Marlatt & Gordon, 1985).

Typically, a fair amount of training is required before a counselor can provide CBT with good adherence to a manual. However, Carroll et al. (2008) developed a computer-based version of CBT that has the potential to drastically reduce training time and expenses. In an initial study, 77 individuals entering a community outpatient program were randomized to receive standard care or standard care plus biweekly access to CBT delivered by a computer, referred to as *computer-based training for CBT* (CBT4CBT). This program consists of six modules, with content taken from Carroll's National Institute on Drug Abuse CBT manual (Carroll, 1998). Material is presented in several formats, including graphic illustration, videotaped examples, verbal instructions and audio voiceovers, interactive assessments, and practice exercises. Results indicated that participants assigned to the CBT4CBT condition submitted fewer drug-positive urine samples over the 8-week trial than those in the standard care condition (mean of 2.2 vs. 4.3) and a lower percentage of drug-positive urine tests (34% vs. 53%); there was also a trend toward longer periods of continuous abstinence (22 vs. 15 days).

Twelve-Step Facilitation

TSF is an individual counseling approach that was designed to help patients engage more fully with 12-step-based self-help programs. This intervention was developed for Project MATCH (Matching Alcohol Treatments to Client Heterogeneity) and used in both the outpatient and aftercare arms of the study (Nowinski, Baker, & Carroll, 1995). TSF takes the patient through the first 5 steps of 12-step programs, which involve acceptance of the self as an addict, surrender to a higher power, and completion of a moral inventory. Other topics include an examination of family history of substance use, learning about situations that lead to substance use, and sober living. Although the National Institute on Alcohol Abuse and Alcoholism has made the TSF manual available, it is not clear how widely this approach is being used.

Marital and Family Therapies

Various kinds of marital and family therapies have been used to provide initial or continuing care for individuals with substance use disorders and their family members. The approach with the most evidence of efficacy is BCT (Epstein & McCrady, 1998; O'Farrell & Fals-Stewart, 2001; Shadish & Baldwin, 2005). Most versions of BCT are focused on both reducing alcohol or drug use in the identified patient and improving overall marital satisfaction for both partners. In BCT sessions, the therapist arranges a daily Sobriety Contract in which the patient states his or her intent not to drink or use drugs that day, and the partner expresses support for the patient's efforts to stay abstinent. The Sobriety Contract can also include urine drug screens for the patient, attendance at other agreed-to counseling sessions, or 12-step meetings by the patient and partner (e.g., Alanon or Naranon); these behaviors are also marked on the calendar and reviewed at each session. The calendar provides an ongoing record of progress that is rewarded verbally at each session. To improve relationship functioning, BCT uses a series of behavioral assignments to increase positive feelings, shared activities, and constructive communication because these relationship factors are conducive to sobriety.

RESULTS FROM STUDIES OF BEHAVIORAL CONTINUING CARE INTERVENTIONS

This section summarizes results from studies of continuing care that have been conducted between the 1970s and 2006. Several studies that have adaptive components are described in more detail in subsequent chapters. The review begins with correlational and quasi-experimental studies of continuing care and then moves to controlled studies. Some of the material presented here has been adapted from previous reviews (McKay, 2001a, 2001b, 2005, 2006).

Correlational and Quasi-Experimental Studies of Continuing Care

Correlational studies that have examined the relationship between participation in continuing care interventions and substance use outcomes have consistently generated positive results. In a review of alcohol aftercare studies conducted before 1985, Ito and Donovan (1986) concluded that greater participation in aftercare was associated with a reduced risk of relapse to heavy drinking, although not necessarily with higher abstinence rates. A review by McKay (2001b) also found that longer stays in continuing care were usually related to better alcohol use outcomes, with some exceptions. For example, veterans who participated in continuing care (i.e., formal aftercare, self-help programs, or both) after residential treatment had better 1-year drinking outcomes than those who did not attend continuing care (Ouimette, Moos, & Finney, 1998). However, veterans who received formal programmatic aftercare only (i.e., no AA attendance) did not have better outcomes than those who did not attend any aftercare or AA.

Longer term participation in AA has also consistently predicted better substance use outcomes. For example, in a sample of individuals with alcohol use disorders who had not received professional treatment, faster affiliation and longer participation with AA predicted better 1- and 8-year alcohol-related outcomes. Individuals who attended AA at least five times per week for the 1st year had an almost 90% likelihood of abstinence at 1 year, and participation in AA had a positive effect on alcohol-related outcomes over and above the effects of formal treatment (Moos & Moos, 2004). The benefits of AA attendance extended out to a 16-year follow-up in this study (Moos & Moos, 2007). Kissin et al. (2003) examined the relationship of attendance at self-help groups and substance use outcomes over 30 months in a large sample of patients who received treatment in publicly funded programs in and around Cleveland, Ohio. Participants were categorized as continuous attendees, starters, stoppers, intermittent attendees, and nonattendees. Results indicated that by the end of the follow-up, rates of substance use were lower in those patients who attended self-help continuously or started to attend during the follow-up, compared with those who attended less regularly or not at all.

The primary limitation of correlational studies is that treatment effects are confounded with various patient characteristics, such as motivation to stop substance use and initial success in treatment. Even controlling for these factors in analyses using newer statistical techniques such as propensity scores does not entirely eliminate the problem. Therefore, only limited inferences regarding causality are possible with such studies. In a quasi-experimental study, participants end up in two or more groups that can be directly compared. However, the participants are not randomly assigned to the conditions, nor are they assigned in some other manner that involves at least some element of chance (e.g., sequential cohort assignment or assigning to second condition when the first condition fills up). Rather, participants self-select into different conditions or are placed in different conditions because of some factor such as severity of drug use.

One quasi-experimental study examined the predictors of participation in step-down continuing care in publicly funded substance abuse treatment programs and the relation between participation in step-down care and alcohol and crack cocaine use outcomes over a 36-month follow-up (McKay, Foltz, et al., 2004). The sample included patients in residential and inpatient programs (IP; n = 134) and IOPs (n = 370) in and around Cleveland. Approximately one third of patients in the IP sample received step-down IOP or standard OP continuing care, and less than a quarter of those in the IOP sample received step-down OP care. Patients who received step-down continuing care following IP had greater social support at intake and were more likely to be female and to be White than those who did not receive continuing care. Patients who received continuing care following IOP were more likely than those who did not to be female and to be employed; they were also older, had higher self-efficacy, and had shorter lengths of stay in IOP. Participation in step-down care was not associated with other factors assessed at intake.

In the IP sample, receiving step-down continuing care was not associated with better alcohol or crack cocaine use outcomes over the 36-month follow-up. In the IOP sample, there were also no main effects favoring continuing care over the whole follow-up period for either alcohol or crack cocaine use outcomes. However, patients who received continuing care did have less crack cocaine use in the first 6 months of the follow-up ($p = .05$), and a trend in the same direction was obtained over the subsequent 6 months (e.g., months 7–12; $p = .07$). In each case, those who received continuing care following IOP reported using cocaine about half as often as those who did not, although the average frequency of use was quite low in both groups.

Koenig et al. (2005) conducted an economic analysis of the benefits of addiction treatment, using data from the same sample that McKay, Foltz, et al. (2004) had studied. Overall, these investigators found substantial economic benefits associated with substance use treatment over a 30-month follow-up, with overall benefit-to-cost ratios of 2.8 to 4.1. Almost all of the benefits came from reduced criminal activity and increased earnings. The economic benefits of the continuum of care were also evaluated by contrasting outcome costs for patients who participated in at least two levels of care (e.g., residential to IOP or OP, IOP to OP) to costs of those who participated in only one level of care. Results indicated that costs for patients who participated in both residential and IOP or OP treatment were approximately 60% lower than costs for those who attended residential treatment only ($p < .01$). However, there were no cost savings associated with attending OP after IOP versus attending IOP only.

Controlled Studies of Continuing Care Treatment Interventions

Literature searches identified 20 controlled studies on the effectiveness of continuing care provided through various behavioral therapies or counseling interventions published since the late 1980s. The results of most of these studies have been summarized in earlier reviews (McKay, 2001a, 2001b, 2005, 2009). These 20 studies are described in Table 3.1. Ten studies included patients with a primary alcohol use disorder diagnosis, whereas the other 10 included patients with drug dependence or a combination of drug and alcohol problems. Participants were graduates of inpatient or residential treatment programs in 12 studies (60%) and graduates of outpatient treatment programs in 5 studies (25%). In the remaining three studies (15%), most participants were graduates of inpatient or residential treatment with a minority from outpatient programs. With regard to study design, 17 studies featured random assignment of patients to two or more conditions. In the other three studies, assignment to treatment condition was done on the basis of sequential cohorts and availability of the experimental condition.

A systematic examination of the methodological rigor of the studies included in this review is beyond the scope of the chapter. However, several comments are in order concerning the study designs. Most of the studies had some strong methodological features. As noted, 17 of 20 studies featured

TABLE 3.1
Controlled Studies of Continuing Care

Citation	Characteristics of subjects	N	Type and duration of CC[a]	Follow-up duration (months)[b]	Main effects
			Studies with negative results		
Gilbert (1988)	Male veterans; alcohol only	96	All subjects received standard aftercare (weekly for 3 months, biweekly for 9 months) and one of three compliance enhancement conditions in first 6 months: none, telephone prompts before session, sessions delivered through home visits	12	CC attendance highest with home visits, and better attendance predicted better substance use outcomes; however, no group differences on five drinking outcome measures
Ito, Donovan, and Hall (1988)	All male; alcohol only	39	8 weekly group sessions: RP vs. interpersonal	6	No group differences on six drinking outcome measures, CC attendance, or change process measures
McLatchie and Lomp (1988)	Alcohol only	155	4 sessions over 3 months, presented as mandatory, voluntary, or delayed 12 weeks	3	No group differences on relapse rate, AA attendance, or other outcomes
				12	Low follow-up rate; data obtained from counselors, not research staff

Study	Sample	N	Treatment	Months	Results
Hawkins, Catalano, Gillmore, and Wells (1989)	82% male; primary drug abusers	130	Skills training and networking activities (2 sessions/week for 26 weeks) + TC vs. TC only	12	Skill level at 12 months higher in experimental condition; marginal effect favoring experimental condition on one of six substance use outcome measures
Cooney, Kadden, Litt, and Getter (1991)	33% women; alcohol only	96	26 weekly group session: coping skills vs. interactional therapy	24	No group differences on heavy drinking days, psychiatric severity, employment, or social behavior
Connors, Tarbox, and Faillace (1992)	68% male; "problem drinkers"	63	Group counseling vs. TEL (8 sessions/calls over 6 months) vs. no aftercare	18	No differences between the three conditions on four drinking outcome measures
Graham, Annis, Brett, and Venesoen (1996)	73% male; alcohol and drugs	192	12 weekly RP sessions: group vs. individual format	12	No group differences on six alcohol or drug use measures; group RP better on social support than individual RP
Schmitz et al. (1997)	50% female; cocaine dependent	32	2 RP sessions/week for 4 weeks vs. 1 session/week for 4 weeks and group vs. individual format	8	No group differences on cocaine urines or time to relapse; some self-report variables favored group format
Project MATCH (1997)	80% male; alcohol only	774	Individual MET, CBT, or TSF (12 weeks duration, with 12 sessions for CBT and TSF, and 4 sessions for MET)	15	No group differences on two primary drinking outcome variables

(continues)

TABLE 3.1

Controlled Studies of Continuing Care   *(Continued)*

Citation	Characteristics of subjects	N	Type and duration of CC[a]	Follow-up duration (months)[b]	Main effects
McKay et al. (1999)	Male veterans; cocaine dependent	132	2 sessions/week for 20 weeks: 12-step-focused group counseling vs. group + individual RP	24	No group differences on frequency of cocaine or heavy drinking days, or on five of six other outcome measures; drinking outcomes in Year 2 favored RP
Studies with positive results					
McAuliffe (1990)	United States: 67% male; Hong Kong: 100% male, 100% Chinese; all opiate addicts	168	RTSH (3 hours/week for 26 weeks) vs. community referrals and/or individual counseling	12	Probability and extent of relapses and level of crime lower in RTSH than control; employment rate higher in RTSH subjects
Foote and Erfurt (1992)	Predominantly male; alcohol and drugs	325	Follow-up contacts (15–24 over 12 months) + standard CC vs. TAU CC only	12	Better outcomes on three substances use–related treatment and cost measures in experimental condition; no differences on three other measures
Patterson, MacPherson, and Brady (1997)	Males; first admissions; alcohol only	127	Nurse visits over 12 months vs. review visits every 6 weeks	60	Higher abstinence rates; fewer blackouts; less gambling in nurse visit group

Study	N	Condition	Population	Months	Findings
O'Farrell, Choquette, and Cutter (1998)	59	15 couples BMT/RP sessions offered over 12 months vs. no CC	Married, male; alcohol only	30	More abstinence days to 18 months and better marital outcomes to 30 months in BMT/RP
Sannibale et al. (2003)	77	Structured aftercare (9 sessions/6 months) vs. unstructured aftercare, sessions provided as requested	Severe alcohol and/or heroin dependent	12	Structured aftercare produced better attendance and lower rates of uncontrolled substance use compared with control
B. S. Brown, O'Grady, Battjes, and Farrell (2004)	194	6 months of aftercare + case management and crisis intervention vs. no further care	Parolees and probationers; 75% male; opiate and cocaine use	6	Aftercare associated with higher rates of abstinence from all drugs, less opiate use, and lower rates of weekly drug use
Horng and Chueh (2004)	68	Five 30- to 60-minute telephone calls over 3 months vs. no further treatment	92% male; Taiwan; alcohol only	3	Higher abstinence rates; better adjustment; lower addiction severity; lower readmission rates in TEL vs. control
McKay, Lynch, et al. (2004) and McKay, Lynch, Shepard, and Pettinati (2005)	359	Group counseling (24 sessions) vs. CBT/RP (24 sessions) vs. TEL (12 TEL sessions, 4 support group sessions)	83% male; cocaine and alcohol dependent	24	TEL produced higher abstinence rates than group counseling and higher rates of cocaine-free urine samples than RP; liver function measures also favored TEL over group counseling and RP
Bennett et al. (2005)	124	Standard care (3 groups/week, social club) vs. SC + Gorski approach to RP (15 sessions)	63% male; abstinent at end of treatment but with history of relapse; alcohol only	12	Lower rates of heavy drinking; fewer drinking days; trend toward higher total abstinence rate in Gorski RP condition, compared with standard care

(continues)

TABLE 3.1
Controlled Studies of Continuing Care *(Continued)*

Citation	Characteristics of subjects	N	Type and duration of CC[a]	Follow-up duration (months)[b]	Main effects
M. D. Godley, Godley, Dennis, Funk, and Passetti (2006)	Adolescents; 71% male; marijuana and alcohol	183	TAU in the community with mixed number of sessions vs. ACC, which included home visits, case management, transportation to employment, and SC (provided over 3 months)	9	ACC participants received more treatment services and had higher marijuana abstinence rates than TAU

Note. From "Effectiveness of Continuing Care Interventions for Substance Abusers: Implications for the Study of Long-Term Treatment Effects," by J. R. McKay, 2001, *Evaluation Review, 25,* pp. 216–220. Copyright 2001 by Sage. Adapted with permission. Also from "Continuing Care Research: What We Have Learned and Where We are Going," by J. R. McKay, 2009, *Journal of Substance Abuse Treatment, 36,* pp. 134–135. Copyright 2009 by Elsevier. Adapted with permission. CC = continuing care; AA = Alcoholics Anonymous; TC = therapeutic community; TEL = telephone-based continuing care; RP = relapse prevention; MET = motivational enhancement therapy; CBT = cognitive–behavioral therapy; TSF = 12-step facilitation; RTSH = recovering training and self-help groups; TAU = treatment as usual; BMT = behavioral marital therapy; ACC = assertive continuing care; SC = standard care.
[a]indicates length of continuing care treatments; refers to planned duration, rather than actual number of sessions attended. [b]Follow-up duration refers to time from baseline interviews, which were usually at the end of the first phase of care or beginning of continuing care.

random assignment of patients to two or more conditions. Follow-up periods were generally long, with 75% of the studies following patients for 8 months or more, and follow-up rates were relatively good. Most studies included widely used measures of alcohol or drug use, which were often confirmed with urine samples or collateral reports. Many studies also went to some length to document adherence to treatment manuals and controlled properly for therapist effects. Although data-analytic approaches varied across studies, most included relevant baseline covariates in the analyses, and some adjusted alpha levels for the number of outcomes examined.

The primary limitation of the studies, from a methodological standpoint, was low power to find group differences, particularly in the studies that did not yield positive findings. The average sample size in studies that failed to yield positive findings was 171 but only 104 with the large Project MATCH (N = 774) taken out of the calculation. Conversely, the average sample size was 164 in studies that did produce positive effects. With a sample size of 104, a treatment effect would need to be relatively large to be statistically significant (Cohen, 1988). More modest effects, although potentially clinically meaningful, would not likely reach statistical significance with sample sizes of 100 or less.

Of the treatments provided in these 20 studies, the most common was some form of cognitive–behavioral treatment (e.g., CBT, skills training, RP), which was provided in 10 studies. The next most common was standard addiction group counseling with a 12-step orientation (5 studies), which was often "treatment as usual" in the clinic or program where the study took place. Other treatments provided in more than 1 study were home visits, interpersonal therapy, and comprehensive interventions. It should be noted that "CBT-like" elements were provided in many of the continuing care treatments that were not pure CBT or coping skills interventions. Most interventions were provided in a treatment setting, although the telephone was used to deliver care in 5 studies.

The studies in Table 3.1 were classified according to whether a positive or negative treatment main effect result was obtained. Studies with positive results were those in which a treatment group difference was obtained on at least one of the primary substance use outcome measures, with no primary outcomes favoring the comparison or control condition(s). Studies with negative results were those in which no treatment group main effects were obtained on the primary substance use outcome measure(s) or mixed results were obtained, such as outcomes on one measure favored one group, whereas the opposite effect was obtained on one or more of the other specified primary substance use outcome measures. According to this classification system, 10 of the 20 studies yielded positive results. Not surprisingly, studies with minimal or no treatment control conditions were somewhat more likely to yield a positive result (7 of 11, or 64%), compared with those with active comparison treatment control conditions (3 of 9, or 33%).

Each of the 10 studies that yielded statistically significant positive results is described in more detail subsequently. However, the fact that a finding is statistically significant does not always indicate that the effect is large enough to be clinically meaningful. One widely used method for judging the magnitude—and therefore the potential clinical significance—of treatment effects is Cohen's d statistic (mean of Treatment A on the outcome measure minus mean of Treatment B, divided by the pooled standard deviation of both means). According to Cohen (1988), a d of 0.20 indicates a small effect, d of 0.50 a medium effect, and d of 0.80 a large effect. Medium effects are usually considered to be of clear clinical significance, although even small effects can be clinically important from a public health standpoint in a large population (West, 2007).

Clinical relevance can also be judged by the difference in proportions of dichotomous outcomes, such as abstinence rates or attendance at any continuing care sessions and the odds ratios that such analyses generate. A recent study published by Miller and Manuel (2008) surveyed clinicians who were participating in the National Institute on Drug Abuse's Clinical Trials Network to determine how large a treatment effect had to be for it to be considered clinically meaningful. These clinicians reported that differences between treatment conditions of 10 to 12 percentage points on dichotomous measures such as total abstinence or a biological indicator of alcohol or drug use were clinically significant.

Studies with positive results are described next in more detail. The clinical significance of the results is addressed through a presentation of effect sizes—when provided by the authors or easily calculated with data included in the report—or of outcomes with clear clinical significance (e.g., differences in rates of abstinence or retention).

Combining Formal Treatment and Self-Help

McAuliffe and Ch'ien (1986) developed a continuing care treatment based on helping addicts learn self-sustaining alternative responses to stimuli previously associated with drug use, primarily through exposure to a community of recovery persons. Their program, which they called Recovery Training and Self-Help, consisted of professionally led recovery training sessions, peer-led self-help styled meetings, and weekend recreational activity. Participants were asked to commit to participating for at least 6 months in the intervention components, and they could continue for up to 1 year. In a randomized study, this intervention was compared with a control condition that consisted of referrals to available continuing care services in the community and crisis intervention counseling from the study staff (McAuliffe, 1990). Participants were opiate-dependent patients who were completing a primary treatment episode, which could have been residential care, detoxification from methadone maintenance, drug-free outpatient counseling, or halfway houses. One of the interesting features of this study was that it was implemented in the United States and Hong Kong.

The primary outcome measure in this study was *favorable outcomes*, which the authors defined as total abstinence or use on less than a monthly basis, coupled with staying out of jail and providing follow-up data. The rates of favorable outcomes in the continuing care condition were 51% and 39% in the first and second 6-month segments, respectively, versus 39% and 25% in each time period in the control condition. The intervention also produced better employment outcomes and self-reported criminal activity outcomes than the control condition. Similar outcomes were generally obtained in the U.S. and Hong Kong samples.

Multimodal Employee Assistance Program Intervention

Foote and Erfurt (1991) compared an extended follow-up procedure that provided up to 24 contacts over a 1-year period with standard follow-up procedures in employee assistance program (EAP) participants who had completed an episode of substance abuse treatment and returned to work. The EAP counselor was located at the workplace, and participants in the experimental condition received an average of 15 contacts over a 1-year period, including seven visits and three telephone calls, compared with an average of 3 contacts for those in the control condition. These contacts were designed to reinforce motivation, address difficulties that had emerged, and arrange for additional care if warranted. The experimental condition produced better outcomes than the standard follow-up procedure on substance abuse treatment costs ($3,623.00 vs. $4,731.00, $p < .05$), number of substance abuse–related hospitalizations (mean of 0.69 vs. 0.81, $p < .10$), and substance abuse disability costs ($385.00 vs. $561.00, $p < .10$), when other relevant variables were controlled. However, these positive effects were relatively small, and substance use outcomes were not assessed in this study.

Home Visits

Patterson et al. (1997) tested the effectiveness of a continuing care protocol that consisted of home visits provided by a psychiatric nurse over a 1-year period. The participants were alcohol-dependent men in treatment for the first time, who had completed a 6-week inpatient program in a rural area. The home visit continuing care protocol consisted of weekly 1- to 2-hour visits for the first 6 weeks and monthly meetings thereafter. When possible, the spouse or other family members were included. Telephone contact was also available for emergencies and advice between visits. The frequency of home visits could be increased following a relapse or other serious problems. The control condition was standard care at the facility, which consisted of review appointments at the hospital every 6 weeks.

Patients in the study were followed for 5 years. Results indicated that those in the home visit continuing care condition had substantially higher rates of continuous abstinence (36% vs. 6%, $p < .001$), were more likely to attend hospital meetings (24% vs. 9%, $p < .05$), and were less likely to report blackouts (36% vs. 55%, $p < .05$) or gambling (26% vs. 45%, $p < .05$). A limitation of this study was that all continuing care was provided by the same nurse, which means that treatment and provider effects were confounded. In addition, assignment to condition was not by randomization; instead, the control condition was provided when the continuing care nurse could not take on new cases (e.g., sick leave, annual leave).

Couples Intervention

O'Farrell, Choquette, and Cutter (1998) studied the effect of providing couples behavioral marital therapy RP sessions to couples who had completed an initial course of BCT. The continuing care condition, which consisted of 15 sessions provided over 12 months, was compared with a no-further-treatment control condition. Fifty-nine couples with an alcoholic husband were randomly assigned to the two conditions, and regular follow-ups were conducted out to 30 months postcompletion of the initial course of BCT.

Results indicated that the continuing care condition produced better drinking outcomes out to 18 months and better marital adjustment out to 30 months, compared with a no continuing care control condition. For example, those receiving RP averaged approximately 94% days of abstinence between months 4 and 18 of the follow-up, compared with about 82% days of abstinence in the control condition, which indicated an approximate 15% increase in days abstinent. In addition, for those alcoholics with more severe drinking and marital problems, the continuing care condition produced better drinking outcomes over the entire 30-month follow-up than the control condition (O'Farrell et al., 1998).

Coping Skills Intervention

Sannibale et al. (2003) evaluated the effectiveness of a structured continuing care program for patients with severe alcohol dependence, heroin dependence, or both who had completed residential treatment. The continuing care intervention (nine sessions over 6 months) was based on a coping skills approach as described by Monti et al. (1989). The control condition was an unstructured approach that provided continuing care counseling sessions when they were requested by the patients. Patients in the control condition who wanted more than one continuing care session had to continue requesting additional sessions.

The structured continuing care intervention produced a fourfold increase in attendance compared with the control condition (odds ratio [OR] = 4.3). However, rates of attendance were quite low in both conditions; the median number of sessions attended was 2 in the structured continuing care condition (range of 1–12) versus 0 in the control condition (range of 0–4). The continuing care condition also produced one third the rate of uncontrolled use of the principal substance of abuse, compared with that in the control condition (OR = .3). The figures describing actual rates of uncontrolled use in each condition were not provided in this report. The conditions did not differ on time to first lapse or first relapse.

Telephone Counseling Intervention

In a small study conducted in Taiwan, graduates of a short-term inpatient stay at a psychiatric center were recruited and assigned to either telephone continuing care or a no treatment control condition. The 30- to 60-minute calls were made in the 1st, 3rd, 5th, 9th, and 13th weeks. During the calls, the therapist provided social support, health care guidance, medical information, and counseling on psychological problems. Results indicated that the telephone continuing care condition produced higher abstinence rates (50% vs. 24%, $p = .02$), better adjustment outcomes ($p < .05$), lower overall problem severity (as assessed by the Addiction Severity Index, $p < .001$), and lower readmission rates (9% vs. 38%, $p < .005$) over a 3-month follow-up than a no continuing care control group (Horng & Chueh, 2004).

Comprehensive Community Reintegration Intervention

The effectiveness of a continuing care intervention for patients in the criminal justice system who had completed outpatient treatment was investigated by B. S. Brown, O'Grady, Battjes, and Farrell (2004). The 6-month treatment was provided at a facility close to the patient's home and was focused on developing and strengthening supports for drug-free living in the community. To that end, the program made use of community organizations and agencies, involved family members, and addressed workplace issues. Services provided included case management, crisis intervention, support for drug-free functioning, skill building, assistance with problem solving, and a peer support group.

Compared with a no-further-treatment control condition, the continuing care intervention produced better outcomes on several key measures. These results were presented with ORs from logistic regression equations. Compared with those in the control condition, participants assigned to receive continuing care had less opiate use (OR = .26, $p < .01$), cocaine use (OR = .36, $p < .05$), any drug use (OR = .37, $p < .01$), and weekly drug use (OR = .20, $p < .01$).

Telephone Plus Group Support Intervention

Our group at the University of Pennsylvania compared two clinic-based continuing care treatments, group counseling, and CBT–RP, with a telephone-based continuing care (TEL) intervention that also included a support group for the first 4 weeks (McKay et al., 2005; McKay, Lynch, et al., 2004). The TEL condition included CBT elements to reduce relapse risk, along with encouragement for and monitoring of the participant's efforts to make use of external supports such as self-help programs. Participants in group counseling were scheduled to receive two group sessions per week, and those in RP were scheduled for one individual CBT–RP session and one group session. Participants in TEL were scheduled for one telephone call per week, which was supplemented with a group session in the first 4 weeks. The participants were all graduates of 4-week IOPs; half were dependent on cocaine and alcohol, 25% on alcohol only, and 25% on cocaine only. The continuing care interventions were provided for 12 weeks, and participants were followed up for 2 years from intake into continuing care.

Results indicated that the telephone condition produced better abstinence outcomes than group counseling and better outcomes than RP on several outcomes (e.g., cocaine urine toxicology, liver function measures indicative of heavy drinking). For example, rates of total abstinence within each 3-month segment of the follow-up averaged approximately 55% in the TEL condition versus approximately 45% in the group counseling condition. Similarly, rates of cocaine-positive urine samples during the follow-up averaged approximately 25% in TEL versus 37% in group counseling (see Figures 8.1 and 8.2 in chap. 8, this volume). Further analyses from this study that examined moderator and mediator effects are described in detail in later chapters.

Relapse Prevention Intervention

A randomized study conducted in the United Kingdom (Bennett et al., 2005) compared standard group-based continuing care with an intervention referred to as Early Warning Signs of Relapse Prevention Training (EWSRPT), developed by Gorski (1995). The participants were alcohol-dependent patients with a history of at least two relapses who had completed a 6-week day-treatment program. The EWSRPT protocol is similar to cognitive–behavioral RP in several respects but places more emphasis on identifying and addressing early signs of vulnerability to relapse, which under the Gorski model is a process that often unfolds over several weeks. EWSRPT was delivered through up to 15 individual sessions by counselors who had been trained and certified in this approach.

Patients in the EWSRPT condition had a lower probability of drinking heavily over the 12-month follow-up than those in the standard condition (26% vs. 45%, OR = .43, p = .04, r = .20). The authors reported an additional statistic, number needed to treat to prevent one relapse during a 1-year period, which was 5. The EWSRPT intervention also produced fewer percentage days drinking (p = .05, Cohen's d = 0.34) and fewer percentage days of heavy drinking (p = .04, d = 0.31). Although the intervention also generated higher rates of abstinence from all drinking during the follow-up than the control condition (31% vs. 17%), this difference did not reach statistical significance (p = .08).

Comprehensive Intervention for Adolescents

M. D. Godley, Godley, Dennis, Funk, and Passetti (2006) randomly assigned 183 adolescents who had completed at least 7 days of residential treatment for chemical dependency to two types of continuing care. The first condition was usual care, which consisted of referral to traditional intensive outpatient and standard outpatient treatment programs in the area. These programs varied considerably in the frequency and intensity of their adolescent services, ranging from one therapy session per week to several hours of services per day, 5 days a week. The experimental condition was referred to as *assertive continuing care* (ACC). ACC combined case management with home visits and a version of the community reinforcement approach, adapted for adolescents (S. H. Godley, Godley, Karvinen, & Slown, 2001). This comprehensive intervention includes a functional analysis of substance use behaviors and skills training in a variety of areas including prorecovery activities, RP, problem solving, communication, and so forth.

Results indicated that adolescents in the ACC condition were more likely to be successfully linked to continuing care services than those in the control condition and received considerably more treatment, case management, and family services. For example, 94% of those receiving ACC were linked to continuing care versus 54% of those in the control condition, which qualifies as a large effect ($p < .001$, $d = 1.07$). Patients who received ACC were also significantly more likely to remain abstinent from marijuana over the 9-month follow-up than those in the control condition (41% vs. 26%, $p < .05$, $d = 0.32$). Outcomes on other substance use measures such use of alcohol and use of any substances also favored ACC over the control condition, but the results were not significant. One of the unique features of this study is that at the time of this writing it is the only published experimental test of an adolescent continuing care intervention.

CONCLUSION

As noted earlier, half of the studies reviewed in this chapter found significant continuing care effects. Should this be taken as evidence that the glass is half empty or half full? One way to evaluate the meaning of this 50% success rate would be to conduct a meta-analysis, which would yield an estimate of the average magnitude and statistical significance of the differences between experimental and control conditions. However, such an analysis is most appropriate with studies that compare an active intervention to a placebo control or minimal intervention and are similar with regard to other aspects of methods, procedures, and design (McKay, 2009). In the studies in this review, almost half compared two or more active treatments. Furthermore, the studies had notable differences in design and procedures. Therefore, a meta-analysis is probably not yet justified, given the state of the literature at this point. However, a careful examination of patterns in the results suggests that a few trends are evident and that certain factors appear to differentiate studies that found significant effects on key outcomes from those that did not.

Year of Publication

It appears that continuing care interventions, or some other aspects of study design or methodology, are improving. Results from the studies summarized in Table 3.1 indicate that none of the continuing care studies focused on alcohol patients published before 1997 yielded a significant treatment condition effect, whereas four of five studies published since 1997 did find significant effects. Among the studies that included patients with drug use disorders, two of six studies published before 2000 yielded significant treatment condition effects, whereas all four studies published after 2000 found significant effects. Without a more systematic and detailed review of the methodological features of the studies, it is not possible to determine whether this trend is due to better interventions, better designed studies, or both. However, as was noted earlier, studies that found significant treatment effects had somewhat larger sample sizes than those that did not, when Project MATCH was not included in the sample size calculation (Project MATCH Research Group, 1997).

Duration

Of the studies in which continuing care was provided for a minimum of 12 months, all three studies (100%) yielded significant effects favoring the extended intervention. Of the studies in which continuing care was provided for more than 3 months but less than 12 months, four of nine (44%) yielded significant findings. Finally, of the studies in which 3 or fewer months of continuing care were provided, three of eight (38%) yielded positive effects. A number of additional long-term disease management studies described in later chapters of this book have also yielded positive effects. This suggests that interventions with longer planned durations may have a greater likelihood of producing positive effects, provided that they are also capable of keeping patients engaged. However, randomized studies that directly compare extended versus short versions of the same interventions are needed before any firm conclusions can be drawn regarding the impact of duration. At this point, there are few, if any, such studies in the literature.

It should also be noted that many patients in the studies reviewed in this chapter did not continue to attend treatment sessions for the full period over which they were offered. For example, in the study by Foote and Erfurt (1991), only 29% of the participants in the extended contact group attended the expected number of therapeutic contacts (e.g., between 11 and 24, depending on relapse status). In most of the other studies, participants attended between 50% and 70% of planned continuing care sessions. However, there were some studies with higher rates of participation; for example, patients in the O'Farrell et al. (1998) study attended an average of 14 of 15 planned RP sessions, and those in the M. D. Godley et al. (2006) study attended an average of 12 sessions out of 12 to 15 sessions that could have been attended.

Intensity

Among the continuing care studies reviewed, there appears to be a weak effect favoring more intensive interventions. Studies that yielded positive effects for more intensive interventions included the study of Gorski's EWSRPT (Bennett et al., 2005), the structured continuing care model developed by Sannibale et al. (2003), the B. S. Brown et al. (2004) intervention for criminal justice patients, and the Assertive Aftercare model for adolescents developed by M. D. Godley et al. (2006). However, several studies either found no effects in comparisons of more versus less intensive continuing care (Hawkins, Catalano, Gillmore, & Wells, 1989; Project MATCH Research Group, 1997), or even effects favoring less intensive continuing care (McKay, Lynch, Shepard, & Pettinati, 2005). It is possible that intensity effects are moderated by other factors, such as duration of the treatment, method of service delivery, and the severity of the patient population.

Method of Delivering Services

One of the notable similarities between interventions that were 12 months or longer is that none of them relied on patients simply to show up at a treatment clinic week after week. Rather, each approach involved taking the intervention to the patient, by involving a spouse, visiting the home, or using the telephone to deliver the intervention. Other effective approaches to the management of addiction, described in subsequent chapters of this book, have also relied on active efforts to locate patients or to bring the treatment to the patients (Dennis et al., 2003; Morgenstern et al., 2006).

Theoretical Approach of Continuing Care

Most of the 10 studies that generated positive findings either tested a variant of CBT or contained elements of CBT. However, many of the 10 studies that did not yield positive findings also evaluated CBT or CBT-like interventions. Therefore, the presence or absence of CBT components did not appear to strongly influence the effectiveness of the continuing care interventions. This finding is consistent with recent reviews that have concluded that CBT does not appear to be more effective than other active and well-delivered interventions in the treatment of alcohol and drug use disorders (Longabaugh & Morgenstern, 1999; Morgenstern & McKay, 2007). No other theoretical approach was represented in enough studies to draw any conclusions regarding relative effectiveness.

Rates of Participation

In most of the randomized studies reviewed here, most participants received more than a few sessions of continuing care, and some received 10 or more contacts. However, in some of the more naturalistic studies, rates of participation in continuing care were much lower (McKay, 2001a). For example, in the examination of continuing care in and around Cleveland (McKay, Foltz, et al., 2004), only one third of those who graduated from residential care and less than 25% of those in IOP received any continuing care. These lower rates of participation are distressingly similar to national data from SAMHSA (2008), in which the median length of stay in IOP was 46 days and only 36% of admissions completed treatment. Clearly, there is a need to develop continuing care interventions that promote sustained retention. Adaptive treatments, which are more flexible and can accommodate patient preference may be one solution to the retention problem.

Magnitude of Effects in Studies With Positive Results

The 10 studies that produced positive effects favoring a continuing care intervention varied considerably with regard to the magnitude of these effects. For example, studies by Foote and Erfurt (1991), McAuliffe (1990), and McKay, Lynch, et al. (2005) appeared to produce relatively small effects, at least on some of the outcome measures. However, the magnitude of the treatment group differences on dichotomous outcome measures observed in the latter two of these studies clearly met the bar for clinical significance established by Miller and Manuel (2008). The difference between the continuing care and control condition of around 12 percentage points on percentage days abstinent in the O'Farrell et al. (1998) study at first glance also seemed to indicate a relatively small effect. However, the study actually yielded a moderate effect according to Cohen's d because of the relatively small standard deviations on the outcome measure. Other studies in this group generated effects with clear clinical significance, such as substantial increases in rates of abstinence, decreases in alcohol and drug use, and increases in linkage to and in attendance at continuing care, compared with control conditions.

Variability of Patient Response

Finally, the actual data from the studies reviewed here suggest that in the majority of studies, approximately one third of patients had good outcomes (e.g., sustained attendance in continuing care and high abstinence rates during follow-up), another third had mixed outcomes, and the final third did poorly (e.g., little or no continuing care participation, low rates of abstinence). Even in studies that produced significant treatment effects, considerable variability of response is still evident in the effective intervention. High variability could reflect a number of factors, including differences in pretreatment substance use severity, co-occurring problems, motivation, or treatment preferences. In addition, most of these treatments were designed to be delivered in a consistent and fixed fashion, regardless of how patients responded. The potential advantages of flexible, or adaptive, continuing care treatment protocols that directly address variability in response are discussed throughout the rest of this book.

Limitations of the Research Reviewed in This Chapter

In many treatment programs, there is now less of a clear demarcation between each phase, or level, of care. This is largely because of the shift to a primarily outpatient service delivery system in which the difference between IOP and OP is smaller than the difference between inpatient or residential care and outpatient care. However, this shift also reflects increasing concern that offering continuing care only to those patients who complete the first phase of treatment may not be the most effective method for managing substance use disorders. In fact, the patients who drop out early from residential care or IOP may be the very patients who could most use a continuing care approach to manage their care in a more effective and cost-effective manner. One of the major limitations of the studies reviewed in this chapter is that almost all focused only on graduates of the initial phase of care. As subsequent chapters of this book demonstrate, many newer approaches to continuing care either enroll patients before they complete their first phase of treatment or they even enroll them in a comprehensive extended program at the point of intake to treatment.

Another limitation of the studies reviewed in this chapter is that the research does not shed any light on how continuing care works—in other words, the factors that mediate or explain how the intervention promotes sustained improvements in alcohol or drug use. Research on mediation effects and other research designed to identify the active ingredients of continuing care is presented in chapter 4 of this volume. As the findings in this chapter have suggested, one important mechanism of action in accounting for the positive effects of continuing care may be longer durations of contact between patients and treatment providers. Accordingly, chapter 4 also reviews a number of studies that have looked at ways to increase retention in continuing care programs.

4

THE THERAPEUTIC PROCESS AND PARTICIPATION IN CONTINUING CARE

In the field of addiction treatment research, researchers are often in the position of not really being able to explain the positive effects obtained in their studies. Most evidence-based treatments are also theory-based—at least to some degree. However, tests of the mechanisms of action suggested by the theories on which the interventions are based often do not yield positive results (Morgenstern & Longabaugh, 2000; Morgenstern & McKay, 2007). Some theorists have argued that positive treatment effects are due primarily to what are referred to as *general therapeutic factors*, such as an empathic and caring therapist and the structure and support provided by regularly scheduled treatment sessions over a prolonged period of time (Baskin, Tierney, Minami, & Wampold, 2003; Wampold, 2001).

However, others continue to assert that particular therapeutic interventions have specific mechanisms of action that influence outcome above and beyond the effects of general factors (DeRubeis, Brotman, & Gibbons, 2005). For example, there is evidence that positive effects on substance use outcomes from 12-step facilitation (TSF) therapy are in fact mediated by the intervention's effect on participation in self-help meetings. Patients who receive this intervention go to more meetings than those who receive other interventions; attendance at the meetings predicts better outcome; and factoring in attendance in the analysis of treatment group effects accounts for a significant amount of the variance in that effect (Longabaugh & Wirtz, 2001). Hence, mediation by a specific effect has been demonstrated, at least for one intervention.

This chapter reviews what is known about the processes and mechanisms of action that appear to account for the positive effects obtained in studies of continuing care. This work includes studies of potential mediation effects, within-session interactions between therapists and patients that are associated with outcome, and correlates of retention and methods to increase retention. This chapter highlights innovative research programs by Karno and Longabaugh on within-session therapeutic processes and by Lash and colleagues on methods to increase retention in continuing care.

STUDIES OF MEDIATION IN CONTINUING CARE INTERVENTIONS

The study of mediation processes in continuing care interventions is still a relatively new area of research in the addictions. The few studies that have been published in this area have generated mixed results. Comprehensive analyses of hypothesized mediators and causal models within the treatment and aftercare arms of Project MATCH (Matching Alcohol Treatments to Client Heterogeneity) were described in a monograph by Longabaugh and Wirtz (2001). The lack of differences in outcome between cognitive–behavioral therapy (CBT), motivational enhancement therapy (MET), and TSF in the aftercare arm effectively curtailed the search for mediation effects (i.e., there were no treatment effects to mediate). However, other hypothesized causal chains linking process variables to outcomes that did not rely on the need for significant treatment group effects also were generally not supported by these analyses.

Conversely, a study that compared relapse prevention (RP) and TSF continuing care interventions yielded some evidence of hypothesized specific therapy effects within each intervention (T. Brown, Seraganian, Tremblay, & Annis, 2002). In this study, there were once again no significant treatment group effects on outcome. However, RP produced higher confidence in one's ability to avoid relapse (i.e., self-efficacy) and lower temptation to drink scores than did TSF at the end of continuing care, whereas there was a trend toward higher scores on a measure of 12-step involvement in TSF, relative to RP. These differences were no longer present at a 6-month follow-up. Further analyses indicated some specificity between treatment process measures and outcomes. For example, changes in self-help involvement predicted drinking outcomes in TSF but not RP, whereas changes in confidence and temptations predicted outcomes in RP but not TSF. Treatment Group × Process Measure interactions also predicted outcomes at 6 months, although the results were inconsistent (i.e., change over different periods predicted different outcome measures) and were found with only two of the five outcomes examined. The lack of a treatment group main effect on outcome precluded a full analysis of mediation effects. Other limitations of this study included a low follow-up rate (approximately 50%) and a lack of clear evidence that the changes in process variables predicted subsequent drinking outcomes.

In a second study of mechanisms of action in continuing care, Mensinger, Lynch, Ten Have, and McKay (2007) used data from the McKay, Lynch, Shepard, and Pettinati (2005) study to conduct mediational analyses to explore how telephone continuing care achieves a positive therapeutic effect. In this study, the telephone continuing care protocol placed considerable emphasis on the patient being the primary agent of change, with less reliance on either a counselor or fellow group members. This message was driven home directly in the content of the intervention and indirectly by the reduced contact with both counselors and group members relative to RP and standard group counseling. In fact, patients engaging in telephone-based continuing care (TEL) had less than half the average minutes of contact with their counselors than did patients in group counseling or RP.

Therefore, the working assumption that directed the search for therapeutic mechanisms of action was that the TEL condition may have prompted patients to make better use of their own internal resources as well as external resources other than the counselor and group members. This assumption generated predictions involving five potential mediator variables. First, the TEL condition was hypothesized to produce better improvements in self-efficacy, commitment to abstinence, and self-help beliefs than the group counseling condition. Second, the TEL condition was hypothesized to produce better improvements on self-help involvement and general social support than the group counseling condition. The analyses examined scores on the mediators at end of treatment (e.g., 3 months) and again at 6 months and controlled for the baseline value of the mediator as well as substance use in the period between baseline and when the mediator was assessed. This was done to adjust for the possible effect of within-treatment substance use on the mediators. The outcome measure was abstinence status assessed within each 3-month segment of the follow-up, after the point at which the mediator was measured.

The mediation analyses yielded support for several of the predictions. First, the TEL condition did sustain higher levels of self-help involvement during treatment than the group counseling condition (i.e., baseline to the 3-month assessment). Self-help involvement at 3 months was in turn a significant predictor of abstinence status between Months 4 and 24. Several further tests for mediation effects recommended by MacKinnon, Lockwood,

Hoffman, West, and Sheets (2002) produced evidence of a significant mediation effect. Second, the TEL condition produced greater increases in both self-efficacy and commitment to abstinence between baseline and the 6-month assessment point than the group counseling condition, and both these variables predicted subsequent abstinence status (i.e., between Months 7 and 24). Once again, further analyses indicated that there were significant mediation effects with both variables (Mensinger et al., 2007).

Overall, these results suggest that initially the greater therapeutic effect of the telephone condition compared with the standard group counseling approach is partially accounted for by a differential change in behavior. Namely, telephone participants indicated more involvement in self-help meetings and related activities during the period of the intervention than their group counseling counterparts. This led to better early posttreatment abstinence outcomes and concurrent increases in self-efficacy and rates of commitment to recovery, which in turn mediated subsequent abstinence outcomes. Therefore, the treatment first yields behavior differences, which are followed by differences in efficacy beliefs and motivation. These results are generally in agreement with models in the addictions (Marlatt & Gordon, 1985) and other areas (Bandura, 1991) in which successful coping (i.e., behavior change) is thought to produce increases in self-efficacy and support commitment to behavior change.

The T. Brown et al. (2002) and Mensinger et al. (2007) studies yielded similar findings with regard to the importance of self-efficacy and how best to increase it. In both studies, the intervention that was more focused on increasing active coping—CBT in the Brown study and TEL in the Mensinger study—produced higher self-efficacy than the comparison condition, and higher self-efficacy in turn predicted better substance use outcomes. However, the studies yielded opposite results regarding the mediating effects of self-help behaviors. In the Brown study, the TSF intervention produced greater self-help involvement than CBT, whereas in the Mensinger study, the TEL intervention led to greater self-help involvement than standard group counseling, which had a strong 12-step orientation. In the latter study, both treatment conditions stressed self-help involvement, but the individual counseling provided in TEL made it possible to keep closer track of whether the patient was indeed going to self-help meetings and to address failure to do so. This may have been more effective than the approach taken in the group counseling sessions.

STUDIES OF WITHIN-SESSION THERAPEUTIC PROCESSES

Using data from therapy sessions in the aftercare arm of Project MATCH (1997), Karno and Longabaugh conducted an elegant series of studies on the impact of therapist counseling style, and the interaction between counseling style and patient characteristics, on drinking outcomes. These studies have also sought to explain the matching effects that were observed in Project MATCH. This work has involved the careful coding of therapist and patient behaviors during treatment sessions for factors such as focus on emotional material, directness, and reactance. These studies have yielded effects in the moderate to large range, making them some of the larger effects obtained in Project MATCH.

The first study examined whether the degree to which therapists focused on emotional material in the treatment sessions interacted with level of depression to predict drinking outcomes. In this study, Karno and Longabaugh (2003) were testing two competing theoretical positions regarding the best way to help depressed patients with alcohol problems. One approach asserts that directly addressing depressed mood and helping patients to cope with depression might reduce the likelihood of relapse, particularly that related to mood. The second approach suggests that focusing on the painful affect might further upset the patient, thereby increasing the risk of relapse.

Results indicated that there was a significant interaction between depressive symptoms assessed at baseline and therapist focus on emotional material in the treatment sessions that predicted drinking frequency and severity over the 1st year of the follow-up. Specifically, patients with clinically elevated depression scores had better drinking outcomes if their therapists had a low focus on painful emotional material and worse outcomes when the therapist focused to a greater degree on such material. Therapist focus on emotional material was not predictive of drinking outcomes in patients who were not depressed. These results therefore supported the latter theoretical position regarding how best to address depressed mood.

Next, Karno and Longabaugh (2004) examined whether degree of therapist directiveness accounted for the moderator effect in Project MATCH, in which MET was more effective than CBT or TSF for patients high in anger. Directiveness was operationalized as the degree to which the therapist employed confrontation, interpretation, and closed-ended questions; addressed in-session resistance; initiated topics; and provided information. Results from analyses performed with patients from the aftercare arm of Project MATCH indicated that higher therapist directiveness predicted worse drinking outcomes in high-anger patients and better drinking outcomes in low-anger patients. Moreover, there was some evidence that therapist directiveness partially mediated the treatment effect favoring MET over CBT for high-anger patients.

Karno and Longabaugh (2005b) also examined whether therapist directiveness interacted with patient reactance to predict drinking outcomes. In this study, *reactance* was defined as the patient's tendency to resist giving up control in interpersonal situations, which in psychotherapy research has been associated with resistance to change. Patient reactance was assessed by coding patient statements and behaviors from the first treatment session. The results indicated that there was a significant interaction between therapist directiveness and patient reactance, which predicted drinking frequency and intensity over the 1st year of the follow-up. Specifically, higher therapist directiveness predicted worse drinking outcomes in patients with moderate or high levels of reactance but was not related to drinking outcomes in those with low reactance. Further analyses indicated that the both interactions (i.e., Therapist Directiveness × Patient Anger and Therapist Directiveness × Patient Reactance) made unique contributions to the prediction of frequency and intensity of drinking outcomes (Karno & Longabaugh, 2005a).

CONTINUING CARE RETENTION STUDIES

A number of studies have focused on identifying factors that are associated with retention in continuing care and methods that can be used to increase engagement with and extended participation in continuing care. Some of the interventions that have been studied include incentives for patients and counselors, behavioral contracting, and intensive referral and linkage.

Correlational and Quasi-Experimental Retention Studies

Several correlational studies have examined potential predictors of participation in continuing care, including demographic factors, substance use severity, co-occurring problems, continuity of care practices, living situation, and distance from continuing care facilities. Harris, McKellar, Moos, Schaefer, and Cronkite (2006) used the Andersen model of help seeking (Andersen, 1995) to identify potential predictors of engagement in continuing care. The participants in the study were 3,000 patients from 15 geographically diverse Veterans Affairs Medical Center (VAMC) residential addiction treatment programs. Variables were selected to represent each domain in the model: predisposing characteristics, need-based characteristics, recovery resources and barriers, and treatment characteristics. Analyses indicated that eight variables were positively associated with a higher number of consecutive months of continuing care following residential treatment: being African American, more pretreatment substance use disorder outpatient visits, higher substance-related problems, a recent suicide attempt, active motivation for change, better cognitive functioning, religious beliefs and behaviors, and a supportive treatment environment. In addition, lower alcohol use frequency before treatment predicted longer stays in continuing care.

Schaefer, Ingudomnukul, Harris, and Cronkite (2005) found that greater use of continuity of care practices by counselors and case managers during outpatient treatment predicted longer participation in subsequent continuing care. Specifically, greater efforts to coordinate care, connect the patient to resources, and provide continuity (i.e., retain same counselors or case managers in continuing care) predicted longer participation in continuing care, whereas efforts to maintain contact with patients after they left the first phase of treatment did not. Notably, continuity of care practices during residential treatment, in contrast to outpatient treatment, did not predict retention in continuing care.

Hitchcock, Stainback, and Roque (1995) studied the relation of patients' living situations while they were in continuing care to retention in continuing care. Results indicated that patients who were living in halfway or recovery houses had better retention and showed greater progress toward the goals of continuing care than those living in other forms of housing in the community. Schmitt, Phibbs, and Piette (2003) found that patients who lived within 10 miles of a continuing care facility were 2.6 times more likely to seek treatment there following discharge from residential treatment than those who lived at least 50 miles from the facility.

Finally, Shepard et al. (2006) attempted to increase retention rates in the middle of a study with patients receiving drug-free outpatient continuing care following residential treatment in a publicly funded clinic. Most of the participants were heroin dependent and had extensive criminal records. When retention rates in the first part of the study proved to be unacceptably low, these investigators began to offer counselors an additional $100 bonus for each of their patients who attended at least five sessions of continuing care. After the incentives were provided, the proportion of patients who attended at least one session of continuing care increased from 64% to 87% (odds ratio [OR] = 4.2, $p < .02$) and the proportion who achieved the five-session milestone increased from 33% to 59% (OR = 4.1, $p = .001$).

These studies suggest that two general factors appear to be associated with better retention in continuing care. First, patients who have a combination of greater problem severity but stronger motivation and greater recovery capital (i.e., social support, supportive living, participation in other prorecovery activities) are likely to be retained longer. Second, situations in which continuing care is either more convenient or more actively encouraged by treatment staff are also likely to promote longer stays in continuing care.

Experimental Retention Studies

Other studies have used experimental methods to test treatment enhancements designed to increase rates of entrance to and sustained participation in continuing care. These include case management, low-cost incentives and active referral, intensive self-help referral, active outreach, telephone encouragement, higher cost incentives, and multicomponent enhancements.

Case Management

The impact of case management on continuing care participation was examined in drug-dependent patients at a VAMC (Siegal, Li, & Rapp, 2002).

Patients were randomized to receive standard primary and continuing care treatment or standard treatment plus case management delivered during both primary and continuing care phases. Patients in the case management condition attended approximately 43% more continuing care sessions than those in standard care.

Low-Cost Incentives and Active Referral

Chutuape, Katz, and Stitzer (2001) were interested in increasing the rates of successful transitions from brief inpatient detoxification to outpatient continuing care. These investigators randomly assigned patients completing a 3-day detoxification to one of three conditions: (a) standard referral to continuing care, (b) referral plus an incentive for completing continuing care intake procedures on the day of discharge from the detoxification program ($13), and (c) incentives plus staff escort to the continuing care program. Rates of completed continuing care intakes were 24% in the standard condition, 44% in the condition with incentives, and 76% in the condition with incentives and a staff escort.

Intensive Self-Help Referral

Many addiction treatment programs have onsite Alcoholics Anonymous (AA) or Narcotics Anonymous self-help meetings that patients attend while in treatment, and virtually all treatment programs refer patients to self-help programs as a form of continuing care following discharge. However, many patients either do not attend at all once they leave treatment or go for only brief periods. Timko, DeBenedetti, and Billow (2006) conducted a study to determine whether more intensive referral to self-help groups during outpatient treatment would promote higher and more sustained rates of participation and better outcomes than standard clinic practices.

The intensive referral intervention was delivered over the first three treatment sessions to patients receiving standard outpatient addiction treatment in a VAMC facility. The intervention consisted of detailed lists of local self-help meetings that had been favored by prior patients, directions to the meetings, and material that described self-help meetings and addressed common questions and typical concerns about the program. The counselor also arranged a meeting between the patient and a participating member of a self-help group and provided the patient with a journal to record attendance at meetings and reactions to the meetings. Attendance at self-help meetings was monitored over the following two outpatient sessions. For patients who had attended a self-help meeting, attempts were made to link the patient with a sponsor. For those who had not attended a meeting, the process of linking the patients with a self-help volunteer was repeated.

Results indicated that patients in the intensive referral condition had higher rates of overall involvement in self-help programs at 6 months than those in the standard referral condition. These patients were more likely to be doing service work at meetings, to have reported having had a "spiritual awakening," to have a sponsor, and to have worked on more of the steps in the 12-step program. However, the effect for overall involvement was small in magnitude ($d = 0.20$), and there was no difference between the conditions in the number of meetings attended. Interestingly, the intervention was more effective with patients who were not heavily involved with self-help in the 6 months before treatment. Specifically, in patients who were below the 75 percentile on prior 12-step attendance, the intensive referral intervention produced higher rates of attendance at self-help meetings than standard referral (62.3 vs. 40.4 meetings during the 6-month follow-up; $p < .01$). With regard to substance use outcomes, the intensive referral condition produced better alcohol and drug use outcomes at 6 months, as assessed by Addiction Severity Index composite scores, and higher rates of total abstinence from drugs than the standard referral condition (Timko et al., 2006).

Active Outreach

Coviello, Zanis, Wesnoski, and Alterman (2006) tested the effectiveness of outreach case management for postdischarge methadone patients. In this study, 128 out-of-treatment heroin users who had been discharged from a program 90 days earlier and were now using drugs again were randomly assigned to receive either a passive referral (PR) for drug treatment or provided with 6 weeks of outreach case management (OCM), a telephone-based intervention designed to help motivate and coach patients to reenter treatment. At 6 months postbaseline, 29% of the OCM participants had successfully reenrolled in drug treatment compared with 8% of the PR participants ($p = .006$). A logistic regression analysis showed that OCM participants were nearly 6 times more likely than PR participants to reengage in methadone maintenance (OR = 5.8, $p = .008$). Moreover, OCM subjects had fewer opiate- and cocaine-positive urine tests at the 6-month follow-up compared with PR subjects.

Telephone Encouragement

A multisite study conducted within the National Institute on Drug Abuse's Clinical Trials Network tested the effectiveness of a telephone procedure designed to increase participation in continuing care following discharge from inpatient programs (Hubbard et al., 2007). Participants were randomized to receive or not receive up to seven brief telephone calls, at 1, 2, 4, 6, 8, 10, and 12 weeks. The role of the telephone counselor was to provide encouragement to comply with the continuing care plan, including attendance at outpatient addiction counseling, participation in AA, and attendance at any other services that were recommended to the patient. Of those in the telephone condition, the average number of calls received was four, and 92% received at least one call. Those receiving calls had a greater likelihood of attending continuing care than those in the control condition (48%

vs. 37%, respectively, $p < .03$), with attendance documented by program records. However, the investigators deemed this a nonsignificant difference after adjusting the significance level for the number of statistical tests performed. These other tests showed no difference between the groups on self-reported alcohol or drug use or attendance at self-help (all assessed at a 3-month follow-up). The relatively small effects in this study may reflect that although the calls provided encouragement to patients, no actual counseling was done.

Higher Value Incentives

In a study at the University of Pennsylvania, we looked at whether CBT and a contingency management (CM) intervention would promote better long-term retention and cocaine use outcomes when used as relapse prevention interventions in patients who had already achieved abstinence in treatment. The CM intervention provided positive reinforcement for co-caine-free urine samples collected three times per week for 12 weeks, in the form of gift certificates for goods or services consistent with recovery or for payment of bills. The value of the reinforcement increased with the number of consecutive cocaine-free urine samples provided; participants could earn as much as $1,150 if they provided 36 cocaine-free samples during the study.

The study participants were 100 cocaine-dependent patients who had been abstinent an average of 45 days and had achieved initial engagement in a publicly funded intensive outpatient program (IOP), as indicated by attending for at least 2 weeks. These individuals were randomly assigned to one of four conditions: IOP treatment as usual (TAU), TAU plus a 12-week escalating voucher reinforcement schedule contingent on cocaine-free urine samples (CM), TAU plus individual CBT-based relapse prevention sessions for up to 20 weeks (RP), or TAU plus vouchers and RP (CM + RP). In the CM + RP condition, patients had to attend their RP sessions to be eligible for the CM procedure that week. Research follow-ups, which included the collection of urine samples and Timeline Followback (L. C. Sobell, Maisto, Sobell, & Cooper, 1979) reports of cocaine use, were conducted at 3-month intervals over an 18-month period.

The total number of IOP group sessions received by participants was 38 in the TAU, CM, and CM + RP conditions and 25 in the RP condition. Therefore, RP, CM, and the combination of CM + RP did not lead to greater participation in IOP. However, the opportunity to participate in the CM procedure did have a large effect on participation in RP; participants in the CM + RP condition attended 13 RP sessions, whereas those in the RP condition attended only three RP sessions ($p < .001$; McKay, Lynch, Coviello, Morrison, & Dackis, 2008).

Cocaine use outcomes were also examined in this study. There were main effects favoring incentives over no incentives on both cocaine urine toxicology and self-report outcomes. These effects were largely accounted for by the CM + RP condition, which had significantly better outcomes than the combination of the other three conditions. Post hoc analyses indicated that the differences between CM + RP and the other three conditions were significant at 6 and 9 months (McKay, Lynch, Coviello, et al., 2008).

Although formal mediation analyses have not been conducted yet, these results suggest that the CM procedure was instrumental in encouraging abstinent IOP patients who had been in treatment for several weeks to attend individual RP continuing care sessions. In fact, the average number of RP sessions attended in the CM + RP group was exactly one session longer than the CM protocol. Further, it was the combination of CM and RP that produced the best cocaine use outcomes. Notably, the benefits of the combined CM + RP intervention persisted for at least 6 months after the end of the CM procedure and 4 months after the end of the RP protocol.

Multicomponent Protocol

Lash, Burden, and Fearer (2007) have been conducting a systematic program of research aimed at increasing attendance in continuing care. The techniques this group has examined include contracts, prompts, and low-cost social reinforcements for attending continuing care. In the contracting procedures, patients are provided with information on the success rates of patients who do and do not attend continuing care (based on prior studies) and are asked to commit to participate in a specified amount of continuing care and other supports (e.g., AA, individual therapy). In some studies, patients are recontracted for a second period of continuing care attendance. Prompts consist of letters from therapists, appointment cards, automated telephone reminders for continuing care appointments, and letters and personal telephone calls following any missed continuing care sessions. The social reinforcement consists of personal letters from counselors with congratulations for attending sessions, certificates for completion of treatment milestones (e.g., 90 days of treatment), and medallions for attending specified numbers of continuing care sessions. The certificates and medallions are typically presented in front of other patients in the therapy groups.

In a first study (Lash, 1998), 40 patients in an inpatient program were randomly assigned either to receive or not receive a 20-minute aftercare orientation session, which included a contract to attend aftercare. Patients who got the orientation were almost twice as likely to attend aftercare as the control condition (70% vs. 40%), and they attended twice as many aftercare sessions (mean of 3.0 vs. 1.4). In a second study, Lash and Blosser (1999) tested the effect of adding attendance feedback and prompts to the aftercare orientation and contract intervention tested in the first study. Results indicated that patients who received the attendance feedback and prompts in addition to the aftercare orientation and contract were more likely to attend aftercare (100% vs. 70%) and attended more aftercare sessions (mean of 4.38 vs. 2.35, $p < .02$, $d = 0.80$) than those who received the orientation and contract only, and they also had fewer hospital readmissions (5 in 21 participants vs. 15 in 20 participants).

Next, Lash, Petersen, O'Connor, and Lehmann (2001) studied whether providing social reinforcement on top of the other intervention components (e.g., orientation, contracting, prompting, feedback) further improved outcomes. To avoid biases that would be caused by randomly assigning patients to both conditions within the same treatment program at the same time, the investigators used an A–B quasi-experimental design. The standard intervention was provided to 43 patients, and then the next 38 patients received the enhanced intervention. The condition that included social reinforcement produced better attendance at aftercare groups over a 12-week period (7.2 vs. 5.2 sessions attended, $d = 0.56$). A second study ($N = 40$) with the same design indicated that patients who received social reinforcement were twice as likely as those in the comparison condition to attend aftercare for at least 2 months (80% vs. 40%, $p = .01$) and had better scores on several other measures of aftercare participation. Moreover, the intervention that included social reinforcement produced higher rates of abstinence at 6 months, as well as better alcohol use outcomes, than the active control condition (Lash, Burden, Monteleone, & Lehmann, 2004).

Most recently, Lash, Stephens, et al. (2007) tested an enhanced version of their intervention, which they refer to as Contracting, Prompting, and Reinforcing (CPR). This enhanced version is extended out for 1 year and targets self-help group attendance as well as aftercare participation. In this study, 150 graduates of a VAMC residential program were randomly assigned to the full CPR intervention, as described earlier, or an aftercare referral-as-usual control condition. Unlike Lash's prior studies, the experimental condition was compared with a more minimal control, rather than to the full package minus one or two components. Therefore, this most recent study was not a dismantling study. Results indicated that patients in the CPR condition were more likely to complete at least 3 months of aftercare (55% vs. 36%), remained in treatment longer (5.5 vs. 4.4 months), and were more likely to be abstinent at 12 months (57% vs. 37%) than those in standard care (Lash, Stephens, et al., 2007).

The work of Lash and colleagues is notable in several respects. First, they have conducted a careful and systematic program of research in which the potential additive effect of each new component of the CPR intervention was determined by testing a version of CPR that included that component against a version that included all other components but not the new component. Therefore, there is empirical evidence for each component of the intervention. Second, the intervention is relatively low cost and can be added to TAU, of any sort, relatively easily. The primary additional burden to the treatment program appears to be time spent by counselors in writing personalized notes and letters to patients at several points during their participation in continuing care.

CONCLUSION

High rates of dropout are a major concern in addiction treatment and are certainly a problem in continuing care. However, the results presented in this chapter indicate that we actually know a fair amount about how to increase retention rates in traditional forms of continuing care. The evidence-based interventions include the following:

- monetary incentives for patients, counselors, or both;
- other types of incentives, such as social recognition;
- personally "handing off" patients from one level of care to the next;
- developing behavioral contracts with patients that specify attendance in continuing care; and
- providing active outreach to patients in the form of case management, linkage to self-help, telephone contacts, and so forth.

These interventions typically produced moderate to large effects that were clearly of clinical significance. One of the other hopeful conclusions that can be drawn from this body of work is that little things matter. The work of Lash et al. (2007), Chutuape et al. (2001), Coviello et al. (2006), and Shepard et al. (2006) suggests that engagement and retention in continuing care can be increased with relatively low-cost, low-effort approaches, which can be applied to virtually any continuing care protocol. This points to the potential benefit of conducting research to identify evidence-based practices and procedures that are easily exported, in addition to the continued search for evidence-based continuing care treatments.

We know comparatively less about why continuing care works. Only a few studies of mediation effects in continuing care have been conducted, and most of these have been hamstrung by a lack of actual treatment group effects to explain. The T. Brown et al. (2002) and Mensinger et al. (2007) studies both found some evidence that confidence in being able to cope without relapsing accounted for some percentage of outcome variance in treatments that directly attempted to improve coping. However, the same effect was not found in Project MATCH. In contrast, the work of Karno and Longabaugh—again using data from Project MATCH—strongly suggests that within-session interactions of therapist and patient factors might shed considerable light on the processes that facilitate or inhibit effective continuing care. Although research that involves the painstaking coding of the content of therapy sessions is arduous and time-consuming, it may be an excellent source for hypotheses concerning the therapeutic process in continuing care (McKay, 2007).

The research described in this and the previous chapter has generally focused on traditional treatment models in which patients transitioned from a relatively brief and intensive initial phase of care to a continuing care intervention that provided treatment of lower intensity and frequency. In some cases, this transition also involved moving from one facility to another, such as when patients enter continuing care in their community after receiving residential treatment at some other location. The next chapter describes newer continuing care models that strive to better integrate successive phases of treatment across the recovery process, in some cases with less of a distinction between each phase.

5

NEW MODELS OF
EXTENDED TREATMENT

The 1st decade of the 21st century has seen the development of a number of treatment models in the addictions that blur the distinction between initial treatment and continuing care. These models, all of which provide extended treatment, make use of innovative strategies to sustain engagement and active participation in interventions to improve management of substance use disorders over time. Another notable feature of several of these care models is that they provide treatment services outside standard specialty care settings. The alternative sites and methods of treatment delivery include visits to primary care offices, use of supportive housing, and monitoring with telephone calls. In addition, some studies have featured extended use of medications.

EXTENDED BEHAVIORAL TREATMENTS

Several investigators have conducted innovative studies looking at the impact of extended models of treatment that include specialized services for

Portions of this chapter have been adapted from "Is There a Case for Extended Interventions for Alcohol and Drug Use Disorders?" by J. R. McKay, 2005, *Addiction, 100*, pp. 1598–1601. Copyright 2005 by Blackwell. Adapted with permission.

specific drug-dependent populations, such as homeless drug addicts, those with severe employment problems, women receiving welfare, and methamphetamine abusers. These interventions have included work therapy and housing contingent on abstinence; intensive case management; and comprehensive behavioral interventions that combine group, individual, and conjoint sessions.

Silverman, Robles, Mudric, Bigelow, and Stitzer (2004) studied the impact of two 12-month behavioral augmentations to standard care for patients who continued to use cocaine regularly during their first 10 weeks on methadone maintenance. Both conditions involved reinforcing cocaine- and opiate-free urine samples by providing take-home methadone doses or a combination of take-home methadone doses and vouchers totaling as much as $5,800, which could be redeemed for goods and services consistent with a prorecovery lifestyle.

Both conditions increased cocaine abstinence during the intervention period, compared with the methadone treatment-as-usual control condition, with the largest and most sustained abstinence in the voucher reinforcement condition. For example, the rate of cocaine- and opiate-free urine samples averaged approximately 60% across the 12-month follow-up in the voucher condition versus approximately 35% in the take-home condition and 15% in the standard care condition. Moreover, the percentage of participants with 100% cocaine- and opiate-free urine samples reached as high as 40% in the voucher condition versus approximately 5% in both the take-home and standard care conditions. The positive effects in the voucher condition persisted during a 9-week postintervention period in those who had completed 12 months of treatment.

In another study of extended treatment, Silverman et al. (2002) evaluated the impact of a long-term, therapeutic workplace in a sample of 40 unemployed, heroin- and cocaine-dependent young mothers on methadone maintenance. The intervention featured the opportunity for full-time employment as a data-entry clerk, and reinforcement was provided for abstinence, attendance, punctuality, professional demeanor, and learning and productivity. The comparison condition was usual care only (i.e., methadone maintenance). Of the 20 women randomized to the therapeutic workplace condition, half maintained steady employment for the majority of 36 months. The percentages of cocaine- and opiate-free urine samples obtained across the entire 36-month follow-up were significantly higher in the therapeutic workplace condition than in the comparison condition (cocaine: 54% vs. 28%, $p = .04$; opiate: 60% vs. 37%, $p = .05$).

Milby and colleagues at the University of Alabama have been conducting a research program on effective interventions for homeless individuals with substance use disorders, most of whom were dependent on crack cocaine. The interventions developed by this group consist of several phases and include housing and work therapy, both contingent on abstinence, as indicated by drug-free urine samples (Milby et al., 1996). The first phase consisted of 2 months of day treatment (i.e., approximately 5 hours/day, 5 days/week), during which lunch and transportation to shelters was provided. Phase II, 4 months in duration, was focused on work therapy, with continued treatment participation at a reduced level. The work therapy involved renovating dilapidated and condemned houses, which in turn were used by the program as drug-free managed housing. Participation in work and access to housing were both contingent on drug-free urine samples. Following a drug-positive urine test, participants could return to work and regain access to housing after providing two consecutive drug-free urine samples.

The first study by this group found that compared with standard outpatient care, the enhanced day-hospital intervention produced less cocaine use, less alcohol use, and less homelessness (Milby et al., 1996). For example, the rate of cocaine-positive urine toxicology samples at 2 months was approximately 30% in the enhanced condition versus more than 60% in the control condition. The effects for alcohol use and homelessness were sustained across the 12-month follow-up, whereas the effects for cocaine use were greatest at 2 months and steadily declined at 6 and 12 months. The enhanced condition also produced a 20-percentage-point increase in percentage of sessions attended (48.4% vs. 28.5%).

In a second study (Milby et al., 2000), the group modified its enhanced day-treatment intervention by moving up access to rent-free housing to Phase I (i.e., first 8 weeks of treatment). Participants qualified for housing after providing four consecutive drug-free urine samples. Phase II was also extended from 4 to 6 months. The work therapy again consisted of housing renovation, under the supervision of the Bad Boy Builders construction company or of food service positions. The control condition in this second study consisted of the day-hospital program only, which was a more intensive intervention than the control condition in the first study.

Results out to 6 months indicated that participants in the enhanced condition attended more treatment activities, had more days abstinent at 2 and 6 months, had higher abstinence rates in each week of the follow-up, and had more days housed at 6 months. For example, rates of urine toxicology–confirmed abstinence were higher in the enhanced condition than the day-hospital-only condition at both 2 (71% vs. 41%, $p < .0001$) and 6 (41% vs. 15%, $p = .0009$) months. The enhanced condition also produced better outcomes on several other drug use measures, including longest period of consecutive abstinence. The enhanced condition averaged 4.9 weeks of consecutive abstinence by the 2-month point versus 2.8 weeks in intensive outpatient program (IOP) only ($p = .0004$, $d = 0.74$). By 6 months, the enhanced condition averaged 9.5 weeks of consecutive abstinence versus 3.9 weeks in IOP only ($p = .0001$, $d = 1.06$). As was the case in the first study, however, the treatment effect on abstinence was no longer present at 12 months (Milby et al., 2003).

Recently, Milby, Schumacher, Wallace, Freedman, and Vuchinich (2005) investigated the impact of providing housing to homeless substance abusers in treatment. In this study, all participants received the phased treatment program that included day-hospital (Phase I, Months 1–2), work therapy and aftercare groups (Phase II, Months 3–6), and aftercare (Phase III, Months 7–12). Participants were randomized into one of three conditions: no housing, abstinence-contingent housing (ACH), and nonabstinence-contingent housing (NACH). Results indicated that participants in ACH and NACH had higher abstinence rates than those in the no-housing condition, with no differences between the ACH and NACH conditions. However, when treatment attendance was controlled, ACH produced higher abstinence rates than NACH. One of the limitations of this study was higher than usual rates of missing urine test data.

Morgenstern et al. (2006) at Rutgers and Columbia studied the effectiveness of an extended, intensive case management intervention in substance-dependent women receiving Temporary Assistance for Needy Families (TANF). In this intervention, case management services were provided for 15 months. Before treatment entry, the case managers met with women at the local welfare office to identify barriers to treatment entry and address resistance to treatment. Plans were developed and implemented to solve child care, transportation, and housing problems, and motivational counseling was provided as needed. Home visits and other outreach activities were also used for women who were having trouble achieving engagement. After the participant entered treatment, the case manager met with her weekly and continued to provide help with coordinating services. Frequency of contact was slowly titrated to twice monthly but could be increased up to daily during crisis periods. Small-value incentives were also provided for attending treatment sessions.

The effectiveness of this intervention was compared with usual outpatient care in a sample of 302 women. Results indicated that the intensive case management intervention produced higher levels of treatment initiation, engagement, and retention compared with usual care. Furthermore, women who received the intensive case management intervention had higher rates of abstinence throughout the follow-up, with the greatest difference obtained at 15 months (43% vs. 26% abstinent). Across the 15-month follow-up, the prevalence of abstinence within each 1-month segment was 75% higher in women who received the case management intervention (odds ratio [OR] = 1.75, p = .025). In a second study of case management, this time conducted in New York City, Morgenstern Hogue, Dauber, Dasaro, and McKay (in press) again found that participants who are provided with case management in addition to treatment as usual (TAU) have better substance use outcomes than those who receive TAU only.

Rawson et al. (1995) at the University of California—Los Angeles developed a phased treatment intervention for stimulant-dependent individuals. This intervention, which is now known as the Matrix Model, consists of two primary phases. The model places a heavy emphasis on individual counseling but also includes a considerable number of conjoint and group therapy sessions, as well as education sessions. In Phase I (Months 1–6), patients receive 20 individual sessions, 16 educational sessions, and 7 conjoint sessions with a significant other and undergo weekly urine testing. Patients also receive a stabilization group for the first 2 weeks and a relapse prevention group thereafter. The program includes a weekly, on-site Alcoholics Anonymous (AA) meeting, and participation in self-help is stressed. In Phase II (Months 7–12), a weekly support group is provided, and individual and couples therapy are available as needed.

Most of the original studies of the Matrix Model indicated that it was associated with reductions in stimulant use, but these studies were not controlled (Rawson et al., 1995). The first controlled study, in which the Matrix Model was compared with other available community resources, examined outcomes out to 12 months. There were no significant treatment group effects on grams of cocaine used, number of cocaine use days, or number of cocaine purchases at 12 months (Rawson et al., 1995). The Matrix Model was recently evaluated again in a multisite study in which methamphetamine (MA)-dependent patients were randomly assigned to receive a 16-week version of the Matrix Model or standard clinic care (Rawson et al., 2004). Results indicated that patients who received the Matrix Model, compared with standard care, attended more treatment sessions, stayed in treatment longer, and had better MA use outcomes (e.g., more MA negative urine samples and longer periods of MA abstinence) during treatment. However, there were no differences between the conditions on measures of drug use or functioning at the end of treatment or at a 6-month follow-up.

Veterans Affairs (VA) has developed a measure of continuity of care that is designed to serve as a performance standard for all Veterans Affairs Medical Center (VAMC) addiction treatment programs. To meet the performance standard, veterans beginning treatment for substance use disorders must maintain continuous treatment involvement for at least 90 days as demonstrated by at least 2 days with visits every 30 days for a total of 90 days in any of the outpatient specialty addiction treatment clinics. It is interesting to note that clinical care by telephone that meets the same standard as face-to-face visits (e.g., staff qualifications, time spent with the veteran) is accepted for continuity of care for visits during the second and third 30-day retention intervals. VAMC programs are rated according to percentage of veterans treated who achieve the continuity of care performance standard. Efforts have been made to establish a mentorship program, which pairs programs with high scores on the performance measure with programs that have low scores in an attempt to provide assistance to these programs and increase the percentage of patients who are retained for at least 90 days.

Initial research on the validity of the VA continuity of care measure has generated mixed results. In a study by Harris, Humphreys, Bowe, Kivlahan, and Finney (in press), up to 50 patients from each of a nationally representative sample of 109 VA substance use disorder (SUD) treatment programs at 73 VA facilities were assessed at intake and posttreatment. In analyses that adjusted for baseline characteristics, meeting the continuity of care performance measure was not associated with patient-level improvements in measures of alcohol or drug use problem severity, days of alcohol intoxication, or days of substance-related problems. However, for the 1,485 patients who were actively drinking or using drugs in the 30 days before entry into treatment, meeting the continuity of care measure was related to significantly increased odds of follow-up abstinence in the propensity score-adjusted analyses (95% confidence interval for OR = 1.27–2.20). These results suggest that drinking and drug use status prior to treatment entry may be a good predictor of whether extended treatment should be recommended.

EXTENDED TELEPHONE MONITORING

One recent trend in addiction treatment is a movement within the traditional, Minnesota model residential rehabilitation programs toward the adoption of a continuum of care approach. Two examples of this new trend are the Betty Ford Center in California and Caron Treatment Centers in Pennsylvania. These programs provide intensive treatment, usually ranging from 28 days to as long as 3 months. Before patients leave the facility to return home, a continuing care plan is developed, which typically includes referral to outpatient treatment, the names and numbers of "alumni" in the area, and contacts with self-help groups. However, leadership at these residential programs became concerned when outcome data suggested that many patients were not following through with their continuing care arrangements as planned.

In response to this concern, Betty Ford and Caron developed telephone-based continuing care programs as a method to enhance patient participation in recovery-related activities in their communities (Cacciola et al., 2008). The intervention currently consists of 13 telephone contacts provided over a 12-month period, which are used to monitor patients' progress and provide encouragement, limited recovery coaching, and treatment referrals as needed. At first, the intervention protocol focused primarily on monitoring substance use and participation in self-help programs. However, Betty Ford and Caron worked with investigators at the Treatment Research Center in Philadelphia, Pennsylvania, to expand, improve, and standardize the interventions, which are now referred to as *Focused Continuing Care* (FCC).

The interventions are now built around a more comprehensive assessment that serves as a "recovery checkup" for the patients. The questions in the assessment ask about current participation in addiction treatment, psychiatric symptoms and treatment, exposure to high-risk situations, craving, self-efficacy, any current use of alcohol or drugs, coping efforts, and participation in self-help. The Caron assessment also inquires about family problems and support and other health-related activities, such as exercise. The new assessment format provides more complete information for the treatment programs on how their residential graduates are doing after they return home. However, the primary purpose of the assessment is to facilitate patients' ability to monitor each component of their recoveries in a more systematic fashion, so that they get into the habit of taking stock of their own progress.

The interventions are delivered by staff members who are dedicated to FCC. They have relatively large caseloads—about 200 patients apiece at Caron, for example. The FCC staff members spend time on the residential units, where they meet with patients before they are discharged and participate in various unit activities. These procedures are designed to forge an initial connection between the patients and the FCC staff members with whom they will be working over the following year. Moreover, the FCC staff members' presence on the unit and their involvement in lectures about recovery and aftercare planning serves to drive home the importance of continuing care to the patients.

One of the interesting issues that is still being sorted out by treatment providers and systems is whether program graduates are still considered to be "patients" of the more intensive, initial treatment program while they participate in telephone-based follow-up and support and other forms of extended care. This is particularly relevant if the participant is also currently engaged in another treatment program where he or she lives. This situation raises questions on several levels. With regard to clinical care, who should the patient contact when problems arise—the staff person back at the initial program or the counselor at the local continuing care program? What if the patient provides different information to each program? How would this be discovered? There is a possibility of splitting or triangulation between each program, especially with patients who are not doing well.

A second question concerns who is ethically—not to mention legally—responsible for the patient. For example, if a patient reveals during a telephone contact that she is suicidal or seriously considering harming someone else, is the initial program still responsible for that patient, even after she has left the facility and started outpatient treatment at home? These questions—who should be providing extended continuing care to patients and who is legally responsible for patients after they have left the primary treatment program—are extremely important issues in continuing care and disease management. We revisit them later in this book.

An article by Cacciola et al. (2008) provides an initial look at patient utilization and outcomes of the original FCC program at Betty Ford in 4,094 patients who received the intervention. Patients completed an average of 5.5 (40%) of 14 scheduled calls, 58% completed 5 or more calls, and 85% were participating in FCC 2 months postdischarge or later. There was preliminary evidence that greater participation in FCC in the first few months yielded more positive outcomes later in the follow-up year and that early postdischarge behaviors predicted subsequent outcomes.

EXTENDED INTENSIVE MONITORING OF PHYSICIANS AND OTHER PROFESSIONALS

Physicians with substance use disorders represent a significant concern for the medical profession and for the public. Their treatment is coordinated by state physician health programs (PHPs) and typically features intensive treatment combined with professional support and frequent random drug testing for 5 or more years.

Procedures in PHPs were recently studied by Dupont, McLellan, White, Merlo, and Gold (2009). Direct services generally included the provision of educational programs for all physicians, consultation with hospitals and clinics, initial assessments of referred cases, interventions with participants, and referral for formal evaluation and treatment. In addition, these programs provide long-term monitoring and documentation of contract compliance. All PHPs required total abstinence from use of alcohol and all other drugs of abuse and provided records documenting abstinence and program participation to licensing boards, hospitals, and malpractice carriers who required this information as a condition of continued ability and eligibility to practice medicine.

DuPont et al. (2009) reported that PHPs were uniformly aggressive in the management of relapse to either alcohol or drug use or to noncompliance with program requirements, with prompt reintervention and referral for further evaluation and treatment. Generally, relapse was classified into levels requiring varying intensities of intervention. For example, in some programs, a Level I relapse was defined as purely behavioral noncompliance, as indicated by missing therapy meetings or support groups, dishonesty, and so forth, whereas Level II involved reuse of drugs or alcohol outside the context of medical practice. Level III relapses were more serious, involving drug or alcohol use within the context of clinical practice including possible impairment within the workplace. Level I relapse typically resulted in reevaluation or contract adjustments, Level II resulted in reevaluation and intensification of additional treatment, and Level III relapse was managed as in Level II but also often included a report to the state licensing board, resulting in the possibility of disciplinary action. Regardless of the relapse category, all PHPs appeared to deal with these occurrences rapidly and with meaningful and sustained therapeutic intervention. Therefore, the PHPs clearly were employing adaptive treatment principles in their protocols.

McLellan, Skipper, Campbell, and DuPont (2008) conducted one of the first studies to determine the long-term outcomes of PHP managed care on the substance use and medical care practices of addicted physicians. The study was a retrospective, intent-to-treat evaluation of chart and urine testing records over a 5-year period, in 904 consecutively admitted physicians to 16 state PHPs. Of the 802 physicians in the sample with known outcomes, 19% failed to complete their contracted period of treatment and supervision. In the 647 physicians who completed treatment and resumed practicing, alcohol or drug misuse was detected through urine toxicology testing in 19% of the physicians over 5 years, with only about 20% in the group with a positive test having more than one such test result. At the 5-year point, 79% of the 802 physicians with known outcomes were licensed without restriction and practicing medicine or working in a nonclinical capacity. These findings indicated that addicted physicians managed by PHPs have favorable long-term outcomes and appear to practice safe medical care.

Another follow-up study looked at the long-term outcomes of physicians enrolled in the Washington Physicians Health Program for substance use problems (Domino et al., 2005). Of the 292 individuals in the study, 25% had one or more relapses during the follow-up period, which was as long as 10 years. This rate of relapse is virtually identical to what was observed in the McLellan, Skipper, et al. (2008) study described earlier. Slightly more than half (58%) of those who relapsed did so within the first 2 years of participation in the program, and only 13% of the physicians had their first relapse after 5 years. Of those who relapsed and were followed for another 5 years, 61% were able to return successfully to the practice of medicine. The major predictors of relapse in this group were a family history of a substance use disorder, use of a major opioid, and a co-occurring psychiatric disorder.

EXTENDED SELF-MONITORING

Helzer, Searles, and colleagues at the University of Vermont have conducted a series of studies in which interactive voice response (IVR) was used to obtain daily reports of alcohol use and other factors over periods of 1 year or longer. In these IVR protocols, participants call into a computer system, which prompts them to answer questions regarding alcohol use and other factors via the telephone keypad. Noting the self-monitoring function served by IVR, these researchers speculated that daily reporting of alcohol consumption over an extended period of time might lead to reduced levels of drinking.

To test this hypothesis, a sample of heavy drinkers who were not seeking treatment were recruited for a study of the effects of daily IVR reporting of alcohol use over a 2-year period. The results indicated that reported alcohol use, as indicated by frequency of drinking, drinks per day, and drinks per drinking day, declined by approximately 20% from the 1st to the 2nd year. At least some reductions in drinking were observed in 82% of the participants. Moreover, the effect of reporting seemed to be specific to alcohol use because there were no significant changes in non-alcohol-related measures (Helzer, Badger, Rose, Mongeon, & Searles, 2002). It should be noted that participants were paid a significant amount of money to maintain consistent participation with the IVR system, which raises questions about whether this approach would work in real-world practice, where such incentives are usually not available. In addition, the lack of a control groups precludes drawing firm conclusions regarding the causal role of IVR in reducing drinking.

EXTENDED MEDICAL MONITORING

Lieber, Weiss, Groszmann, Paronetto, and Schenker (2003) studied extended monitoring and counseling for 789 heavy drinkers with significant alcoholic liver disease. The authors reported that patients of this type are usually referred to specialty care addiction treatment programs but rarely go. In this study, patients received comprehensive monthly visits with a nurse and brief visits with a physician for as long as 5 years, with approximately half of the sample participating for at least 2 years. The sessions contained the main elements of brief interventions, including feedback, personal responsibility for change, advice, menu of change options, empathy, and self-efficacy boosters. Participants' average alcohol consumption dropped from 16 drinks per day before enrollment to 2.5 drinks per day thereafter. It is difficult to interpret these results because of the lack of a control group and the high attrition rate. However, the results suggest that extended treatment delivered through visits to a medical service delivery setting may be an effective method for managing patients who have serious medical illnesses in addition to alcohol use disorders.

Willenbring and Olson (1999) conducted an important study that used randomization to test whether a treatment model that provided integrated medical and addiction treatment for alcoholics with severe medical problems would yield better outcomes than standard treatment. The integrated care model, referred to as *integrated outpatient care* (IOT), provided for monthly clinic visits with a nurse practitioner or physician. Biological indicators were used to track the effects of drinking, and data from these indicators were presented to patients in graphic form to illustrate trends over time. Motivational interviewing techniques were used in the sessions, and family members were included when possible to support change and reduce behaviors on the part of family members that may have enabled drinking. Outreach attempts were made to reengage patients who missed sessions. Patients in the control condition received standard care, which consisted of referral to traditional specialty addiction treatment and advice from medical staff to abstain from alcohol.

The results indicated that the integrated care model produced much higher rates of extended participation in both medical and addiction treatment over the 2-year follow-up than standard care. For example, patients in IOT had an average of 42 treatment visits over 2 years versus 17 visits in standard care. IOT also produced better substance use outcomes. At the end of the 2-year follow-up, 74% of IOT patients were abstinent versus only 47% of those in standard care. More patients in standard care died during the 2-year follow-up compared with IOT (30% vs. 18%), although this difference was not statistically significant. The estimated incremental cost of IOT over standard care was about $1,100 per patient per year.

EXTENDED PHARMACOLOGICAL TREATMENTS

Most studies that have evaluated the efficacy of various pharmcotherapies for addiction have tended to be only 8 to 12 weeks in duration, with the exception of studies on methadone. Although these studies can provide information on whether a medication has any short-term effects, they typically yield no information on how patients do when put on the medications for longer periods of time. This is the case even if the study has an extended follow-up after the short dosing period has ended. As McLellan et al. (2005) pointed out, why would one expect to see a treatment effect 6 or 12 months after the intervention had ended, particularly if the intervention had been a medication? The other limitation in many pharmacotherapy studies in the addictions is that the inclusion criteria require that patients are still drinking or using drugs in the week before they begin the study (i.e., have current use). Therefore, these studies are focused on abstinence initiation rather than abstinence maintenance. However, several studies have evaluated extended courses of treatment with medication.

Sees et al. (2000) used an experimental design to compare the results of a 16-month methadone maintenance (MM) protocol with those of a gradual detoxification program that consisted of two phases: 6 months of methadone plus enhanced psychosocial services and an additional 8 months of individual and group therapy (i.e., aftercare). Results indicated that the MM intervention produced better treatment retention (median of 438 vs. 174 days) and lower rates of drug-related HIV risk behaviors than the detoxification condition. Rates of heroin use were also lower in MM during months 5 to 12 than in the detoxification condition. For example, patients in MM used heroin on 5 to 10 fewer days per month, and rates of any heroin use were 15 to 20 percentage points lower. Conversely, there was no difference between the two conditions on employment, family functioning, or alcohol use. These results clearly indicate that sustained MM produces better outcomes than an intervention of comparable total duration but with a shorter time on methadone.

In a study conducted in the VA system (Krystal, Cramer, Krol, & Kirk, 2001), 627 veterans with chronic, severe alcohol dependence who had been abstinent for at least 5 days were randomly assigned to 12 months of naltrexone, 3 months of naltrexone followed by 9 months of placebo, or 12 months of placebo. All patients were offered individual counseling and were encouraged to attend AA meetings. At 52 weeks, there were no significant differences among the three groups in the percentage of days on which drinking occurred and the number of drinks per drinking day. However, a recent reanalysis of this trial indicated that naltrexone doubled the odds of being categorized in an abstainer trajectory versus a consistent drinker trajectory (Gueorguieva et al., 2007).

A recent large-scale, multisite study tested the efficacy of an injectable form of naltrexone for the treatment of alcohol dependence (Garbutt et al., 2005). Patients in the study received a low-intensity psychosocial intervention and one injection per month for 6 months of either 380 milligrams of naltrexone, 190 milligrams of naltrexone, or placebo. The major difference between oral naltrexone and the injectable form is that after a patient receives an injection, the daily decision regarding whether to take the medication is eliminated, and compliance is assured for at least 30 days.

Results indicated that compared with placebo, the larger dose of naltrexone reduced heavy drinking by 25% over the 6-month study period, whereas the smaller dose reduced drinking by 17%. Treatment effects were larger in men than in women. Compliance with the injection schedule was relatively good; approximately 65% of the patients in each condition received all six injections. A follow-up analysis from this study focused on those patients who had 4 or more days of voluntary abstinence before treatment initiation (n = 82). In this group, there were much stronger effects favoring injectable naltrexone over placebo. For example, rates of favorable response were 70% in the naltrexone group versus 30% in the placebo group (p = .006), and median days of any drinking per month was 0.7 in the naltrexone group versus 7.2 in the placebo group (p = .005; O'Malley, Garbutt, Gastfriend, Dong, & Kranzler, 2007).

During the 1990s, the efficacy of acamprosate as a treatment for alcohol dependence was evaluated in 10 studies, most of which were conducted in Europe. Although the action of acamprosate is not entirely clear, it appears the drug functions as a gamma-aminobutyric acid receptor agonist and that it may also lower neuronal excitability by reducing the postsynaptic efficacy of excitatory amino acid neurotransmitters. One of the interesting features of the European studies was that most featured an extended protocol (12 months), which was considerably longer than the typical length of pharmacological trials in the United States. These studies provided strong initial support for acamprosate with regard to decreasing drinking in alcoholics following initial detoxification. Virtually all of these studies generated positive findings during the treatment phase, and some have indicated that the effects of acamprosate persist to some degree in posttreatment follow-up periods (Carmen, Angeles, Ana, & Maria, 2004; O'Brien & McKay, 2006). However, recent studies conducted in the United States have not replicated these initial favorable results (Anton et al., 2006).

Finally, S. M. Hall, Humfleet, Reus, Munoz, and Cullen (2004) compared the efficacy of extended versus short pharmacological and behavioral treatments. Although this study focused on smoking cessation rather than on alcohol or drug use, it is one of the few studies that have directly compared short versus extended versions of the same interventions for the treatment of an addictive disorder. Therefore, the results are clearly informative and may apply to other addictive disorders. In this study, smokers were randomized to one of four treatment conditions in a 2 × 2 design (nortriptyline vs. placebo and short vs. extended treatment). The short treatment groups received 8 weeks of medication, five group counseling sessions, and nicotine patches. Those randomized to the extended conditions received an additional 44 weeks of medication, 9 monthly counseling sessions, and between-session checkup telephone calls.

At the Week 52 follow-up, smoking point-prevalence abstinence rates were highest in the extended nortriptyline condition (50%), followed by the extended placebo condition (42%), the placebo brief treatment condition (30%), and the brief nortriptyline condition (18%). Of note, participants who received extended behavioral treatment without active pharmacotherapy did better than patients who received both medication and behavioral treatment for a short period.

CONCLUSION

Almost all of the controlled studies of extended treatment reviewed in this chapter yielded positive findings. That is, patients who received the extended interventions had better substance use outcomes than those in the control conditions. However, in most studies, the control condition did not consist of a shorter version of the protocol that was used in the extended intervention. Rather, it was generally some form of TAU. Therefore, the treatment effect might well be due to the superiority of the components used in the extended intervention over what was included in standard care, rather than to the amount of time over which these components were provided. However, both the Sees et al. (2000) and S. M. Hall et al. (2004) studies found that extended versions of pharmacological or behavioral treatment produced better outcomes than shorter versions of the same intervention. Other studies had promising results but did not feature control conditions (Helzer et al., 2002; Lieber et al., 2003).

There has been little work on the targeted use of medications at various points in extensive interventions or on the adaptive use of medications in such interventions, at least in substance-dependent individuals (cf. Kranzler, Armeli, Feinn, & Tennen, 2004, and Kranzler et al., 2003, on targeted use of naltrexone with problem drinkers). For example, compliance with extended care might be improved if alcoholic patients who relapse during the post-treatment monitoring phase were given the choice to take a medication such as naltrexone or acamprosate combined with intensified monitoring rather than return to standard outpatient treatment. As more effective medications are developed and better information is available on which patients respond best to which medications, the potential role of pharmacological agents within extended interventions will no doubt be greatly expanded.

A number of interventions that were evaluated in the studies reviewed in this chapter include elements of adaptive interventions. For example, the opportunity to work on a given day in the Silverman et al. (2002, 2004) studies was contingent on having a drug-free urine sample that day. Similarly, access to housing and work in the Milby et al. (1996, 2000, 2003) studies was contingent on drug-free urine samples. In the Morgenstern et al. (2006) study, the frequency of contacts with case managers could be increased during crisis periods. Further, in the physician health programs, noncompliance with treatment or substance use leads to modifications in the treatment protocol and reports to licensing boards. However, some of these studies are not truly adaptive because they lack specific algorithms that tie clearly defined scores on tailoring variables to changes in treatment.

The chapters in this part of the book have traced the evolution of continuing care interventions, from the use of group counseling and AA following residential treatment to much more sophisticated models of continuing care that include features such a incentives, case management, access to housing and employment, and pharmacotherapy. Information on mechanisms of change and methods to improve retention in continuing care was also presented. In Part III, the chapters present information on adaptive models of care and describe studies of adaptive treatment for depression, hypertension, and smoking cessation. The findings of adaptive studies conducted with patients who have substance use disorders are also reviewed in detail.

III

ADAPTIVE TREATMENT MODELS

6

INITIAL ATTEMPTS TO INDIVIDUALIZE TREATMENT FOR SUBSTANCE USE DISORDERS

Adaptive treatment is an approach to individualizing treatment to ensure that each patient receives the most effective type and intensity of care at a given point in time. In addiction treatment, there is a rich tradition of attempting to improve treatment outcomes by matching patients to various types of treatment or additional services on the basis of need and symptom severity at intake. These matching studies represent a type of adaptive treatment, albeit one that is limited to one adaptation based on data obtained at intake or baseline, rather than modifications driven by progress or the lack thereof during treatment.

In this chapter, research on two types of matching is reviewed. The first type, referred to as *patient-by-treatment matching*, attempts to optimize treatment by discovering which types of patients will respond best to which kinds of addiction treatment. An example of this approach is research that determines whether patients with greater dependence severity at intake do better in inpatient or outpatient treatment. The second type of matching involves providing additional treatment enhancements or services on top of standard addiction treatment that are designed to address co-occurring problems. An example of this approach is providing psychiatric services to patients in standard addiction treatment who also have a mood disorder. It should be noted that most of the matching studies reviewed in this chapter have been conducted in the initial phase of treatment rather than at the start of continuing care.

PATIENT-BY-TREATMENT MATCHING

The observation that some individuals seem to profit greatly from addiction treatment whereas others show no apparent benefit dates back to the early days of formal treatment. In fact, the Alcoholics Anonymous (AA) Big Book talks at great length about the fact that many people are not "ready" for AA and are only willing to devote limited efforts (i.e., "half measures") to the program. Consequently, their failure to achieve abstinence and recovery is no surprise. To some extent, treatment researchers have moved past the notion that one is either ready for treatment or not to the position that different types of individuals may require different types of interventions. According to the matching hypothesis, various characteristics of the patient or of his environment, assessed at or near intake to treatment, will indicate what type of addiction treatment will be most effective. Matching studies have typically tried to identify factors that predict success in various intensities (e.g., inpatient vs. outpatient) or types (e.g., interpersonal, cognitive–behavioral therapy [CBT], motivational interviewing [MI]) of treatment.

Level of Care

With regard to treatment intensity, there has been mixed evidence on whether patients with more severe addiction problems will do comparatively better in high-intensity programs than in low-intensity programs. One of the comprehensive systems that has been developed to improve the matching of substance abuse patients to various levels of care is the American Society of Addiction Medicine's (ASAM; 2001) *Patient Placement Criteria*. The ASAM placement system provides guidelines for assessing patients in two medical problem areas (i.e., acute intoxication/withdrawal and physical complications) and four psychosocial problem areas (i.e., emotional/psychiatric complications, treatment acceptance, relapse potential, and recovery environment). Ratings in each of these areas, or *dimensions*, are used to determine the appropriate level of care, ranging from nonintensive outpatient to medically managed intensive inpatient units.

McKay, Cacciola, McLellan, Alterman, and Wirtz (1997) evaluated the predictive validity of the psychosocial components of the ASAM criteria for placement in residential versus intensive outpatient settings. The participants were 292 male veterans with alcohol or cocaine dependence who received either residential or intensive outpatient treatment at Veterans Affairs facilities. The psychosocial dimensions of the ASAM criteria were first operationalized with instruments with demonstrated reliability and validity. The criteria were then used to determine whether patients in inpatient and intensive outpatient rehabilitation programs were correctly matched to the level of care they received. The patients were followed up at 3, 6, and 12 months postrehabilitation, and outcomes of "matched" and "mismatched" patients were compared in a number of ways. Alcohol and cocaine patients who were correctly matched to treatment according to ASAM did not have significantly better outcomes than those who were mismatched. Furthermore, a more focused analysis generated no evidence that alcohol patients who met ASAM criteria for inpatient care had better outcomes in that setting than in intensive outpatient treatment. Among cocaine patients who met ASAM inpatient criteria, inpatient care did produce marginally better short-term outcomes on most measures, although these results were not statistically significant.

However, several recent studies have provided more support for ASAM and ASAM-like matching algorithms. In a study of dual-diagnosis patients, Chen, Barnett, Sempel, and Timko (2006) found that high-severity patients had better alcohol, drug, and psychiatric outcomes when treated in high-intensity program, compared with low-intensity programs. Moderate-severity patients, in contrast, did equally well in both low- and high-intensity programs. Timko and Sempel (2004) reported similar findings in another study of dual-diagnosis patients. Magura et al. (2003) compared patients who were matched versus those who were mismatched according to the ASAM criteria. Patients who qualified for intensive outpatient treatment but received standard outpatient care had poorer drinking outcomes than those who were correctly matched to level of care. Overall, overtreatment did not improve outcomes. Finally, Tiet, Ilgen, Byrnes, Harris, and Finney (2007) found a matching effect such that patients with more severe substance use disorders at intake had better outcomes in residential or inpatient treatment, relative to outpatient care.

In a study done in the 1980s, McLellan et al. (1983) found that psychiatric severity at baseline could be used to match patients to level of care. It is interesting to note that the strongest matching effects were found in patients with middle-level psychiatric severity. Patients with low-level psychiatric severity did well in all treatments, whereas those with high-psychiatric severity did poorly in all treatments. Weisner et al. (2000) set out to replicate this in a study that compared standard outpatient treatment (OP) to day-hospital treatment (DH) in more than 1,000 new admissions to a large HMO's chemical dependency program. Of the study sample, 668 participants were randomized, and another 405 who were either unwilling or unable to be randomized were also followed up. Patients were followed for 8 months, and outcome consisted of self-reports and urine toxicology screens. The results found no main effect differences between standard OP and DH. However, in patients with midlevel Addiction Severity Index (ASI) psychiatric composite scores, those who received DH had better alcohol abstinence outcomes. The results of these two studies suggest that researchers may need to look beyond linear effects to uncover clinically significant matches between patient characteristics and different intensities or types of treatment.

Type of Behavioral Treatment

Recently, Morgenstern and McKay (2007) reviewed the literature on matching effects in several treatments for substance use disorders, including CBT, MI and motivational enhancement therapy (MET), and 12-step facilitation (TSF). In Project MATCH (Matching Alcohol Treatments to Client Heterogeneity; Project MATCH Research Group, 1997), CBT was hypothesized to be superior to MET and TSF for patients with greater psychopathology, sociopathy, and poorer social functioning. Prior to Project MATCH, studies had generally supported these hypotheses for alcohol dependence (Mattson et al., 1994). Overall, findings supported only 1 of 10 matching hypotheses for CBT. A subsequent prospective matching study also failed to support earlier findings that CBT would be differentially effective for those high in psychiatric severity and sociopathy (Kadden, Litt, Cooney, Kabela, & Getter, 2001).

In cocaine-dependent patients, early studies conducted by Carroll and colleagues found that those with higher drug use severity and levels of depression did better with CBT compared with interpersonal therapy or clinical management (Carroll, Nich, & Rounsaville, 1995; Carroll, Rounsaville, & Gawin, 1991). Subsequent studies have failed to confirm that CBT is differentially more effective for patients with greater depression or psychopathology (Crits-Christoph et al., 1999; Rohsenow, Monti, Martin, Michalec, & Abrams, 2000). Two studies also failed to confirm that CBT is more effective for those with greater drug use severity (Maude-Griffin et al., 1998; Rohsenow et al., 2000), and three studies failed to find that antisocial personality disorder moderated effects for CBT (Crits-Christoph et al., 1999; McKay, Alterman, Cacciola, Mulvaney, & O'Brien, 2000; Rohsenow et al., 2000).

With regard to MI and MET, a number of potential moderators that are consistent with the theoretical underpinnings of these interventions have been examined in meta-analyses and in separate studies. Four studies have examined whether MI worked better for patients with low readiness to change—individuals the intervention was specifically designed to reach. MI did produce better substance use outcomes than the comparison condition for patients low in readiness in two studies; results were mixed in one study, and there was no effect in another study (Butler et al., 1999; Heather, 1996; Monti et al., 1999; Project MATCH Research Group, 1997). Miller, Yahne, and Tonigan (2003) also found no evidence that baseline motivation level interacted with treatment condition to predict outcome. Neither the Miller et al. study of MI for drug use disorders nor a cannabis treatment study that included an MI condition (Marijuana Treatment Project Research Group, 2004) found any significant moderator variables.

One moderator effect involving MET was found in data from Project MATCH. Patients from the outpatient sample with high scores on a measure of anger, obtained at baseline, had better drinking outcomes if they received MET rather than CBT or TSF, whereas the opposite was the case for those low in anger (Waldron, Miller, & Tonigan, 2001). However, this effect was not found in the aftercare sample in Project MATCH (Project MATCH Research Group, 1997) and was also not replicated in the Miller et al. (2003) study.

Few studies have tested theory-driven patient-by-treatment matching hypotheses in TSF treatments, and only two positive findings have been identified. Project MATCH tested 12 separate patient-matching hypotheses in which TSF was hypothesized to be superior to CBT, MET, or both. Only two of the hypotheses were supported. TSF was superior to CBT for those high in alcohol dependence and superior to MET for patients with high levels of network support for drinking. Examination of causal chains found full support for one of these finding. TSF resulted in higher levels of AA affiliation, and this led to better outcomes in TSF for those with high network support for drinking (Longabaugh, Wirtz, & Connors, 2001).

A recent study by Witkiewitz, van der Maas, Hufford, and Marlatt (2007) made use of more sophisticated data analytic techniques to revisit the self-efficacy by CBT matching hypothesis that was tested—unsuccessfully—in Project MATCH. These investigators used the Project MATCH data set for their analyses. The statistical methodologies used in this report were catastrophe and two-part growth mixture modeling, which included posttreatment and baseline self-efficacy. These analyses pointed toward a dynamic relation between self-efficacy and alcohol use in which there were nonlinear interactions between baseline self-efficacy and change in self-efficacy over the follow-up in models to predict alcohol use outcomes. The growth mixture analyses suggested that among patients who drank frequently during the follow-up, those with low self-efficacy at baseline had better drinking outcomes in CBT than in MET (by approximately 20%). Conversely, frequent drinkers with high self-efficacy at baseline had better drinking outcomes in MET than in CBT.

Marlowe and colleagues at the Treatment Research Institute in Philadelphia have also generated more positive results in a series of studies on matching amount of judicial supervision provided to drug offenders on the basis of risk factors. This research has been conducted in drug courts, which use attendance in treatment and drug urine screens to monitor the progress of the offenders. In these studies, offenders were randomized to attend status hearings in a drug court on a biweekly basis or on an as-needed basis, which was much less frequent. Marlowe, Festinger, and colleagues found that of-fenders who met *Diagnostic and Statistical Manual of Mental Disorders* (DSM–IV; 4th ed.; American Psychiatric Association, 1994) criteria for antisocial personality disorder or who had a history of prior treatment for drug use dis-orders did better in the biweekly hearing condition, whereas those who did not meet either of these criteria (i.e., the low-risk offenders) actually did better in the as-needed status hearing condition (Festinger et al., 2002). These findings were replicated in a second retrospective design study (Marlowe et al., 2003) and confirmed in a prospective study in which offenders correctly matched to either biweekly or as-needed status hearings did better than those randomly assigned to these two conditions (Marlowe, Festinger, Dugosh, Lee, & Benasutti, 2007).

Matching on the Basis of Genetics

Three recent studies have raised the possibility that genetic factors might be used to match patients to treatments. On the basis of animal and human laboratory data, Oslin et al. (2003) hypothesized that variations in the mu-opioid receptor gene might account for differences in response to the medi-cation naltrexone, which blocks opiate receptors in the brain. Prior research had suggested that in some people, the rewarding effects of alcohol are medi-ated to a greater degree by the endogenous opioid system. In these individu-als, blocking opiate receptors might therefore lead to a greater reduction in the pleasant or euphoric effects of alcohol consumption. These investigators tested this hypothesis by doing secondary analyses of data from three pla-cebo-controlled, randomized studies of naltrexone, focusing on a functional polymorphism of the mu-opioid receptor. The results indicated that the posi-tive effects of naltrexone on drinking outcomes relative to placebo were much stronger in those who had this genetic polymorphism than in those who did not. This effect was replicated in data from the COMBINE study (Anton et al., 2008). Interestingly, this genetic polymorphism associated with better response to naltrexone is not found in people of African descent. So far, there is no published evidence that people of African descent are less likely to respond to naltrexone in clinical trials. Therefore, the polymorphism of the mu-opioid receptor cannot provide a complete explanation for why some people respond to naltrexone but others do not.

A second study made use of data from Project MATCH to investigate genetic predictors of differential treatment response (Bauer et al., 2007). Prior research has suggested that the *GABRA2* gene confers risk of conduct disor-der and alcohol dependence and is associated with electroencephalographic profiles that have been linked to poor outcomes in alcohol- and drug-dependent individuals. In Project MATCH data, the low-risk genotype predicted better drinking outcomes over the follow-up. Moreover, a treatment effect favoring TSF over both CBT and MET on measures of any drinking and heavy drinking emerged when only those participants with the low-risk genotype were considered in the analyses. Conversely, there were no treatment group differences in those who had the high-risk genotype: All three conditions had similarly poorer outcomes. These findings are reminiscent of the results of the Weisner et al. (2000) and McLellan et al. (1983) studies in which matching effects were found in patients with midlevel problem severity, not in those with higher severity.

PROVIDING SERVICES FOR IDENTIFIED PROBLEMS

A second type of matching approach involves providing additional services, which are not considered part of standard addiction treatment, to address specific co-occurring problems in the patient. McLellan and colleagues at the University of Pennsylvania and the Treatment Research Institute conducted a series of studies in the 1990s that investigated whether adding services that address co-occurring psychiatric, family and social, and employment problems to standard substance abuse treatment programs could improve outcomes. The main studies in this research program have been performed in methadone maintenance (McLellan, Arndt, Metzger, Woody, & O'Brien, 1993), employee assistance (EAPs; McLellan et al., 1997), and publicly supported outpatient drug-free (McLellan et al., 1998) programs. The rationale for this approach is that (a) co-occurring problems in these areas have frequently predicted worse treatment outcome in substance abusers and (b) prior research has shown that treatments that address these problems can improve outcomes.

McLellan and colleagues studied two approaches to providing combinations of adjunctive services. In one approach, a set group of services is offered to all participants, regardless of individual problem severity levels. For example, the impact of adding additional, professionally delivered treatment services to a basic methadone program was investigated (McLellan et al., 1993). In this study, patients were randomly assigned to receive (a) methadone only; (b) methadone plus standard counseling; or (c) methadone and counseling plus on-site medical, psychiatric, employment, and family therapy services (the enhanced condition). Improvements in the enhanced condition were significantly greater than those in the methadone plus counseling condition in employment, alcohol use, criminal activity, and psychiatric status.

McLellan and colleagues also evaluated the impact of adding a case manager to coordinate and expedite the use of adjunctive medical, housing, social, and employment services for substance-dependent patients in publicly supported outpatient treatment programs. The results indicated that the case manager condition produced improved substance use, physical and mental health, and social function outcomes at 6 months, relative to standard care (McLellan et al., 1998). Another comprehensive intervention that provides adjunctive services is the community reinforcement approach (CRA; Meyers & Smith, 1995), which includes basic skills training, a job club, social and recreational counseling, access to a substance-free "social club," and marital therapy. Studies have consistently found CRA to be an effective treatment (Miller & Wilbourne, 2002).

The second approach to providing adjunctive services is to match specific services on the basis of problem severity or need at intake, rather than provide the same menu of services to all patients. This approach was tested by McLellan et al. (1997) in two inpatient and two outpatient private treatment facilities used by an EAP. At intake, patients ($N = 130$) were placed in one of the four programs, assessed with the ASI, and randomized to either the standard or matched services conditions. In the standard condition, the treatment program received information from the intake ASI, and personnel were instructed to treat patients as per usual clinic procedures. For patients in the matched services condition, the programs agreed to provide at least three individual sessions in the areas of employment, family and social relations, or psychiatric health delivered by a professionally trained staff person when a patient evidenced a significant degree of impairment in one or more of these areas on the intake ASI. For example, a patient with significant impairments in the areas of social and psychiatric functioning would receive at least six individual sessions—three by a social worker and three by a psychiatrist.

The following results were obtained when the standard and matched conditions were compared over a 6-month follow-up period. First, matched patients received significantly more psychiatric and employment services than standard patients but not more family and social services or alcohol and drug services. Second, matched patients were more likely to complete treatment (93% vs. 81%) and showed more improvement in the areas of employment and psychiatric functioning than the standard patients. Third, although matched and standard patients had sizable and equivalent improvements on most measures of alcohol and drug use, matched patients were less likely to be re-treated for substance abuse problems during the 6-month follow-up. These findings suggest that matching treatment services to adjunctive problems can improve outcomes in key areas and may also be cost-effective by reducing the need for subsequent treatment.

The services to problems studies that have been done by McLellan et al. (1993, 1997, 1998) have also had several important limitations. First, the number of adjunctive treatment sessions provided has been relatively small (e.g., 2–3/area), which may have produced findings that underestimated the potential effects of the intervention. Second, the follow-up periods have generally been short (e.g., 6 months), which raises questions about the durability of the effects. If the purported theoretical underpinnings of the intervention are supported (i.e., the adjunctive services actually reduce comorbid problems and reductions are predictive of better drug use outcomes), then treatment effects should persist and possibly increase over time relative to control conditions.

Friedmann and colleagues conducted a large-scale study of services-to-needs matching that addressed some of the limitations of the work by McLellan and colleagues. This study was conducted with a sample of more than 3,100 addiction treatment patients. The study focused on the degree to which reported needs in five domains—medical, mental health, family, vocational, and housing—were addressed with services and whether better matching produced better substance use outcomes. Overall, higher rates of services-to-problems matching predicted better substance use outcomes. The effect was concentrated in patients who reported problems in more areas (e.g., at least four of the five domains) and was strongest among patients in long-term residential facilities. Matching of vocational and housing services was particularly important (Friedmann, Hendrickson, Gerstein, & Zhang, 2004).

Not all studies of attempts to match services to problems have produced positive effects. One recent quasi-experimental study (Fiorentine, 1998) evaluated whether substance-abusing patients with family, housing, legal, medical, emotional, and vocational problems (a) were more likely to resolve these problems if they got services in those areas and (b) whether resolution of those problems was associated with better substance use outcomes. The results indicated that improvements in these areas were generally not greater in those who received treatment in each area. Improvements in family and housing problems were associated with better in-treatment drug use outcomes, but the resolution of problems in the other areas was not associated with better drug outcomes during treatment or at 6- and 24-month follow-ups. This study therefore generated little evidence that supported the need to treat co-occurring problems.

However, the Fiorentine (1998) study had several major limitations that make it difficult to interpret the findings. First, the sample was restricted to patients who had been enrolled for at least 8 weeks in outpatient treatment. Patients who dropped out earlier, who might have benefited most from adjunctive services, were not included. Second, co-occurring problem severity at baseline was assessed retrospectively at follow-up through self-report. Third, the assessment of problem severity was conducted with only two items per area, rather than with psychometrically validated scales. Finally, the only data obtained on services received in a particular area concerned whether any services had been received (yes–no).

As many practicing addiction counselors and program directors will report, it can be difficult to deliver additional adjunctive services to patients who are already participating in intensive treatment. A recent study by our group can be seen as an example of what can go wrong when attempting to match services to problems. In chapter 5, a study was described in which we evaluated whether adding contingency management or individual CBT sessions for patients who had achieved abstinence in intensive outpatient programs (IOP) improved outcomes (McKay, Lynch, Coviello, Morrison, & Dackis, 2008). Prior to conducting that study, we had performed a similar one that examined the impact of CM and matched services, rather than CBT, in patients recruited in their 1st week of IOP.

During a pilot testing phase for this study, we developed an algorithm to match patients to services. Those who met DSM–IV criteria for depression were eligible for cognitive therapy (CT; Beck, Rush, Shaw, & Emery, 1979), those who had a significant other who was willing and able to participate in conjoint treatment were eligible for behavioral couples therapy (BCT; O'Farrell, Choquette, & Cutter, 1998), and those who wanted assistance with vocational problems were eligible for an intervention designed to improve readiness for work and provide help with job seeking and retention (Metzger, Platt, Zanis, & Fureman, 1992). The algorithm spelled out a procedure for prioritizing need should the patient qualify for more than one service, and it also provided guidance on how patients could be switched to a different type of service, if the problem that was prioritized was resolved. The condition that included matched services and CM was pilot tested in patients who were stably engaged in IOP, and it performed well.

Unfortunately, the adaptive algorithm did not work as well in the actual study. Patients who were just starting in IOP tended to be overwhelmed with the requirements of that program (e.g., approximately 10 hours of group treatment/week) and were not looking for any additional treatment. Many others dropped out of IOP before they could get started with our matched services. Moreover, few patients either met DSM–IV diagnostic criteria for current depression or had a significant other who was willing to participate in BCT and were appropriate for that intervention. Further, as it turned out, the vocational intervention was not well received because the program did not want patients to be too focused on employment issues early on in their recoveries, and the patients themselves had similar feelings (McKay, Lynch, Morrison, & Coviello, 2009).

CONCLUSION

The research findings from studies of patient-by-treatment matching present a mixed picture. There is some evidence that severity of substance use and other co-occurring problems can be used to determine the level of care that is likely to be most effective. Specifically, patients with more severe problems appear to do better in higher levels of care, such as inpatient rather than outpatient treatment, more rather than less frequent judicial supervision, and so forth. However, the replication by Weisner et al. (2000) of a prior study by McLellan et al. (1983) suggests that the relationship between severity and optimal treatment intensity may not always be linear. There is also intriguing research suggesting that genetic factors may be useful for selecting optimal matches to both pharmacological and behavioral treatments. One of the studies suggested that differences in the effectiveness of behavioral interventions might be more likely to emerge in lower risk patients. Conversely, there is much less evidence to indicate that variables measured at intake are useful for matching patients to different behavioral therapies of relatively similar intensity and mode of service delivery. However, several studies have indicated that matching specific adjunctive services to co-occurring problems can improve substance use outcomes (Friedmann et al., 2004; McLellan et al., 1997).

Taken as a whole, these findings suggest that there still may be some life in the matching hypothesis, despite the generally gloomy conclusions engendered by the National Institute on Alcohol Abuse and Alcoholism's Project MATCH (Burhringer, 2006). However, the effects are likely to be small and probably relatively short-lived because of many of the factors discussed in chapter 2. Matching based on information gathered at intake might be compared to a sailor's initial attempts to set the rudder and trim the sails of his boat after he has had a chance to observe wind direction and swell height upon arriving at the harbor. However, these initial settings are likely to change after the boat is out on the ocean because conditions continue to evolve. In addiction treatment research, variables assessed at intake may be significant predictors of response to treatment, but they usually account for only a small percentage of the variance in outcome. The ability to adjust or adapt treatment at one or more points after whatever matching is done at intake is likely to be particularly important in continuing care because patients' symptoms wax and wane over time. In chapter 7, we provide a detailed look at the concept of adaptive treatment and reviews some of the findings on the effectiveness of this approach in other disorders, including depression, hypertension, and smoking cessation. In chapter 8, we review a number of studies of adaptive treatment that have been conducted with patients who have substance use disorders.

7

ADAPTIVE MODELS OF TREATMENT

In the addictions, data from numerous treatment studies indicate that there are large individual differences in patient responsivity, even to effective treatments that have been standardized and with therapists who adhere closely to treatment manuals. It is not unusual, for example, for results in these studies to indicate that approximately 40% of patients complete treatment and achieve abstinence, another 20% attend most sessions but continue to drink or use drugs, and the remaining 40% drop out of treatment early. This important point also applies to treatments that clearly "work" for the majority of people to whom they are delivered because there are always a certain number of nonresponders, even to the most efficacious interventions.

Despite this considerable variation in patient response, most treatments in the addictions strive to deliver essentially the same intervention to all patients, regardless of how the patient is responding. This is particularly the case in carefully controlled research studies. For example, in studies of manualized treatments such as cognitive–behavioral therapy (CBT) or behavioral couples therapy (BCT), patients all progress through a series of modules or components, according to the blueprint laid out in the manual. If a patient is not responding as expected, the protocol may be slowed down a bit, but the intention is still to deliver a full course of CBT or whatever the treatment happens to be. Deviations from the intended course of treatment are seen as problematic. Some protocols do provide opportunities for the patient and therapist to select specific modules from a menu, as was the case in the combined behavioral intervention that was tested in the COMBINE study (Anton et al., 2006). However, in most cases, the opportunities for choice are at the end of the protocol, after all the required modules have been delivered.

As is well known, however, medical care for a wide range of disorders does not adhere to fixed protocols. Rather, physicians change the treatment if a patient is not demonstrating sufficient response. Treatment for hypertension and depression provide good examples of flexible treatment algorithms. In the case of hypertension, patients are usually started out on a medication such as a diuretic, which is effective, inexpensive, and well tolerated by most patients. If response is inadequate or side effects too troublesome, the physician may add a second medication from a different class (e.g., beta blocker) or switch to another medication entirely (e.g., angiotensin-converting enzyme [ACE] inhibitor). Symptom status (i.e., blood pressure) is monitored over time, and further adjustments to the treatment regimen are made as needed. Practice guidelines have been worked out that provide medication algorithms for physicians to follow (ALLHAT Collaborative Research Group, 2002).

In this chapter, the concept of adaptive treatment is more fully introduced, and a case is made that this approach better addresses heterogeneity of response than standard treatment models. Two approaches to developing adaptive treatment algorithms are described, one that makes use of the knowledge or judgment of experienced clinicians and a second that uses experimental procedures to determine optimal algorithms. New developments in methods to derive adaptive algorithms are discussed, including designs in which patients who fail to respond after randomization to an initial intervention can be randomized additional times to further treatment alternatives. Finally, adaptive approaches to the treatment of other diseases are discussed.

ADAPTIVE TREATMENT:
AN ANSWER FOR RESPONSE HETEROGENEITY?

Approaches to the treatment of medical and behavioral disorders in which changes in symptoms or status are monitored over time and used to adjust the treatment protocol according to well-specified guidelines have been labeled *adaptive treatment protocols* (L. M. Collins, Murphy, & Bierman, 2004; Murphy et al., 2007; Murphy & McKay, 2004). These protocols are also known by a number of other names, including *stepped care, treatment algorithms,* and *dynamic treatment regimes* (Lavori, Dawson, & Rush, 2000; Murphy, 2003).

The main components of an adaptive treatment are tailoring variables, therapeutic components or options, and decision rules (L. M. Collins et al.,

2004; Murphy et al., 2007). Tailoring variables are the measures that are used to monitor patient progress. Often, the primary outcome measure, such as alcohol or drug use, is used as a tailoring variable. In that case, changes in treatment might be triggered by failure to stop using cocaine or other drugs during treatment. However, other measures, such as attendance in treatment sessions or self-help groups or scores on measures of self-efficacy or motivation, might also be used as tailoring variables. For example, decisions to increase or decrease the intensity of treatment over time might be driven by changes in the patient's perceived ability to cope with various problems without drinking (i.e., abstinence self-efficacy). Even in the absence of actual drinking, sharp declines in self-efficacy could indicate that a change in treatment is required.

Decision rules are the "if–then" statements that link responses on the tailoring variables to specific changes in therapeutic components or procedures. An example of a decision rule might be, "If the patient has 3 or more heavy drinking days within a 7-day period, augment standard outpatient treatment with individual CBT sessions" or "If blood pressure readings of less than 140/90 are not achieved after 2 weeks on a diuretic, augment with a beta blocker." Decision rules can also be used to step-down treatment from a higher to a lower intensity, such as, "If the patient has achieved 4 consecutive weeks of confirmed abstinence, step down from intensive outpatient treatment to standard outpatient treatment." It should be noted that decision rules are clearly operationalized; they involve specified cutting scores on the tailoring variables and specified treatment selections.

In most cases, adaptive protocols contain separate algorithms for two main classes of patients: nonresponders and responders. The tailoring variable is used to determine whether an individual is responding to the initial treatment provided. There are several possible treatment modifications that could be considered for nonresponders. These options include augmenting treatment by providing something else in addition to the current treatment or switching to an entirely different treatment. In continuing care for addictions, for example, one could augment standard care by adding an additional form of treatment (e.g., adding individual CBT or a medication to group therapy). Examples of switching in the addictions include stepping treatment up to a more intensive level (e.g., outpatient programs [OP] to intensive outpatient program [IOP] or residential care), a lateral move from one type of behavioral therapy to another (e.g., a 12-step-based treatment to CBT), some other modification to the content of the therapy (e.g., emphasis on family issues to other relapse triggers), and changing modality (e.g., behavioral therapy to medication).

In addition, one might consider providing step-down care to a particular group of nonresponders: those who drop out of treatment quickly. A low-level monitoring approach may be advantageous with these patients to facilitate some sort of engagement. It is important to consider the nature of the nonresponse when considering possible treatment modifications. For example, the most effective algorithm would likely recommend different kinds of modifications for nonresponders who keep coming to treatment but continue to use substances than for those who simply stop coming to treatment.

With responders, the task is to identify the point at which the patient can be stepped down to a lower intensity treatment and still maintain good outcomes. Most patients would rather not continue to come to a clinic on a regular basis and would prefer a more convenient, lower burden form of ongoing care. However, stepping a successful patient down too quickly can lead to increased risk of relapse. Moreover, with some disorders, such as diabetes and hypertension, reductions in medication are generally possible only when there are significant and sustained changes in lifestyle factors (e.g., changes in eating habits, frequency of exercise). One important question for the field is whether research can determine standard guidelines that can be applied to all patients (e.g., "Once the patient has achieved 4 weeks of continuous abstinence in IOP, step down to OP"), or whether heterogeneity of patient response will preclude such general guidelines.

METHODS FOR DEVELOPING ADAPTIVE INTERVENTIONS

Adaptive interventions are developed through one of two approaches: one that makes use of existing research and clinical knowledge to craft the algorithm and another that instead relies on experimental procedures to derive optimal combinations of tailoring variables and interventions. Both approaches have been used to develop algorithms for addiction treatment.

Nonexperimental Approaches

The more common approach to developing adaptive interventions is to use a combination of prior research findings, expert consensus, and common sense to derive the treatment algorithm. In the addictions, the American Society of Addiction Medicine's (2001) *Patient Placement Criteria*, discussed in chapter 6 of this volume, is a good example of that approach. These criteria were developed over time by a group of experienced treatment providers and researchers and are widely used by many local providers and state systems to assign patients to an initial level of care. The criteria also provide guidelines for when patients have achieved sufficient progress to be stepped down to a lower level of care. Placement and continuation decisions are derived from algorithms that are based on problem severity levels in six dimensions: acute intoxication/withdrawal, physical complications, emotional/psychiatric complications, treatment acceptance, relapse potential, and recovery environment.

The effectiveness of an adaptive algorithm developed through expert consensus can be evaluated in a randomized trial in which it is compared with standard treatment, another adaptive algorithm, or some other control condition. The main advantage of this approach is that only one randomized study is necessary to determine the effectiveness of the algorithm after it has been developed and pilot tested for feasibility. The main disadvantage is that if the adaptive intervention does not produce better outcomes than the control condition, it will not be clear where the "weak link" is in the algorithm. For example, the problem could be that the wrong tailoring variable was used, that the wrong cutting score on an otherwise appropriate tailoring variable was selected, that the wrong therapy options were included for nonresponders, that there was another problem with the decision rules, or some combination of two or more of these factors.

Experimental Approaches

The other approach to developing adaptive interventions involves the use of experimental designs to determine optimal treatment algorithms (Murphy et al., 2007). For example, there may be some disagreement on when to declare a patient a nonresponder to the first treatment provided. This could be an important issue because keeping a patient on a treatment that is not working could heighten the risk of dropout. However, some treatments, including CBT, appear to show "sleeper effects" (Carroll et al., 1994; McKay et al., 1999), and it would therefore be contraindicated to switch too quickly. One could attempt to arrive at a consensus on the optimal point to declare a patient a nonresponder, through discussions with clinicians and other experts (as described earlier). Or patients could be randomized to two or more definitions of nonresponse and outcomes observed. The definition that produced the best overall outcomes would then be selected for the algorithm. Randomization could also be used to determine the optimal form of treatment for nonresponders to the first treatment provided. In studies designed to develop adaptive pharmacotherapy algorithms for various disorders, a primary consideration with nonresponders is whether to add a second medication (i.e., augment) or stop the original medication and change to a different one (i.e., switch). This can be determined through randomization to each strategy.

Similarly, randomization can be used to compare possible continuation treatments for initial responders. Because the successful management of chronic disorders usually requires adherence to medication and behavior change routines over long periods of time, considerable care must be taken not to overburden patients, so that they continue to be willing to participate appropriately in their treatment. Therefore, it can be advantageous with responders to step down their level of care at some point to ensure their continued participation. Randomization can be used to compare two or more continuation treatments to determine which approach promotes better long-term compliance and sustained reductions in symptom severity.

After an optimized adaptive algorithm is developed through the experimental method, it should be further tested against treatment as usual or some other control condition in a randomized clinical trial. This step is needed to determine whether the algorithm in fact improves outcomes relative to standard care. Unfortunately, this means that it is usually necessary to obtain additional funding and conduct a second study to confirm the effectiveness of the adaptive intervention. Additional information on how to select tailoring variables and construct decision algorithms for adaptive interventions is presented in chapter 10.

Adaptive treatment protocols hold considerable promise for improving the long-term management of alcohol and drug dependence because they are a good match for the clinical course of these disorders. Specifically, individuals with substance use disorders frequently go through periods of abstinence or nonproblematic use after receiving an episode of treatment (Dennis & Scott, 2007; Hser et al., 2007; McKay, 2005; McKay et al., 1999). During these periods, they are not likely to be willing to continue to attend regular face-to-face treatment sessions at a chemical dependency program beyond a few months. However, many of these individuals will eventually engage in problematic drinking or drug use again. At that point, it may be difficult to reach patients who have relapsed and reengage them in treatment. In an adaptive treatment protocol, the level or intensity of treatment is substantially reduced when patients are doing well to relieve burden on the patient, promote greater compliance with treatment, and reduce costs. However, some degree of regular contact is maintained, so that worsening of symptoms or deteriorations in functioning can be caught more quickly and increased frequency or intensity of care arranged when necessary.

As was discussed in chapter 6, efforts to match patients to specific addiction treatments or to additional services on the basis of variables assessed at intake to treatment have produced mixed results. Adaptive treatment also represents an attempt to match specific treatments to individual patients. What, then, is the justification for this approach given the failure to obtain stronger and more consistent results with other matching approaches? The key difference between adaptive treatment approaches and the more traditional patient-by-treatment matching approach is that the former makes use of information on response to treatment, in addition to or instead of intake data, to guide the selection of further treatment, whereas the latter relies on intake data only.

NEW DEVELOPMENTS IN ADAPTIVE TREATMENT

Adaptive protocols developed under the first approach described earlier (e.g., expert consensus, literature reviews) may have multiple branches in the treatment algorithm. For example, an algorithm might state, "Start with Treatment A; if patient fails to respond, switch to Treatment B; if patient fails to respond, add Treatment C to Treatment B," and so forth. Similarly complicated protocols can also be developed through the experimental approach. However, this requires randomizing patients two or more times, which is referred to as *sequential randomization*.

A relatively new development in adaptive treatment is the use of sequential multiple-assignment randomized trials (SMARTs; L. M. Collins, Murphy, & Strecher, 2007; Lavori & Dawson, 2004; Murphy, 2005; Murphy et al., 2007; Ten Have, Joffe, & Cary, 2003) to build and refine adaptive treatment strategies with multiple decision points. These designs yield a number of algorithms that can be compared on various outcome measures to determine which algorithm produces the best overall outcomes. For example, a SMART study with two randomization points and two treatment options at each randomization point will generate eight algorithms consisting of various combinations of if–then statements. Each algorithm provides comprehensive directions regarding how to tailor interventions to individual patients. In the data analyses of such a study, the algorithm that produces the best overall outcomes is identified. An example of a SMART study with two randomization points is provided in chapter 9.

One of the advantages of SMART studies is that it is possible to examine the impact of the later decision points while taking into consideration earlier decision points. For example, the effectiveness of a particular continuation treatment for initial responders may depend on what the initial treatment was. Similarly, the effectiveness of a particular step-up treatment for nonresponders may depend on the criteria for declaring someone a nonresponder. If separate studies are performed for each randomization point, these kinds of interactions cannot be examined.

The major disadvantage of SMART studies concerns the potential implications for sample sizes. Even with only two randomizations, there are many possible comparisons, and the number of participants in each algorithm can be small unless the overall sample size is relatively large. One way to address this is to specify in advance the most important comparisons. Typically, certain hypotheses are considered primary, whereas others are relegated to secondary status. Stronger inferences are possible with results generated by the primary hypotheses. Results from the secondary analyses are considered hypothesis generating and can be confirmed in subsequent studies. Another issue that results from these designs is the need for care in determining the effect of early randomizations. These issues are discussed further in chapter 11.

A second development in the field is the inclusion of patient choice, or preference, in adaptive algorithms. In an adaptive protocol that includes patient choice, the selection of the next treatment is not governed completely by randomization. Rather, patients may be randomized to a condition in which they can select one of two or three options versus a condition that does not include choice. The incorporation of patient preference or choice is increasingly seen as crucial to effective medical care (Krahn & Naglie, 2008). However, choice may be particularly important in the addictions, in which patients often declare themselves as nonresponders by dropping out of treatment rather than by continuing to attend while still drinking or using drugs. For example, patients with alcohol use disorders who do not become engaged in standard abstinence-oriented outpatient treatment within 2 weeks of intake might be offered a choice of several other treatment approaches (e.g., medication, telephone monitoring, CBT).

Providing patients with a menu of possible treatment options may improve rates of sustained engagement and participation. However, it poses a number of problems for researchers. First, it creates heterogeneous treatment conditions in research studies; in other words, different patients in the same condition get different interventions. If such a condition yields better outcomes than a comparison condition, the effect might be because patients had a choice or it could be due to the superiority of the particular option that was chosen more frequently. If the latter is the case, it may be more important to provide that particular treatment to all patients than to offer a choice that includes the treatment. Unfortunately, the only way to determine this is to do a second study, in which the menu of treatment options is compared with the one treatment from the menu thought to be most effective.

Building choice into an adaptive treatment study makes an already complicated study design all the more daunting, especially if the study features sequential random assignment (i.e., a SMART study). In such a study design, the researcher is likely to end up with small sample sizes in some groups, unless the study sample is substantial. If some of those conditions include multiple treatment options, interpretation of results can become difficult. These issues are discussed in more detail in chapter 11.

EXAMPLES OF ADAPTIVE TREATMENT IN OTHER DISORDERS

At this point, adaptive or stepped care treatment algorithms have been developed and evaluated for a number of disorders, including depression and anxiety (Otto, Pollack, & Maki, 2000; Scogin, Hanson, & Welsh, 2003; van Straten, Tiemens, Hakkaart, Nolen, & Donker, 2006), obesity and eating disorders (Carels et al., 2005; Wilson, Vitousek, & Loeb, 2000), hypertension (ALLHAT Collaborative Research Group, 2002), and breast cancer screening (Clark et al., 2002; Rakowski et al., 2003). Here, we take a detailed look at four such studies. The first was a large-scale effort to develop an algorithm to treat depression, with a focus on pharmacotherapy (Sequenced Treatment Alternatives to Relieve Depression [STAR*D]; Rush et al., 2004). It is by far the most ambitious and complicated adaptive study that has been performed to date. The second study evaluated a stepped care algorithm for the treatment of hypertension (ALLHAT Collaborative Research Group, 2002). The third study tested an algorithm that used regular assessments of patients' progress in psychotherapy to help therapists adjust treatment over time (Lambert, Hansen, & Finch, 2001; Lambert, Whipple, et al., 2001). The final example is a study that tested a computerized algorithm used to tailor smoking cessation messages (Strecher et al., 2005).

Sequenced Treatment Alternatives to Relieve Depression

One of the key questions in treatment for depression is what to do with patients who do not respond to an initial medication. Should their initial medication be switched to something else? If so, what? Or should they receive another medication to augment what they are already taking? Although practicing psychiatrists have developed their own algorithms to address the issue of nonresponse, the field had not generated an empirically supported set of tailoring variables and decision rules specifying the medication that is most likely to be effective in the face of initial nonresponse.

These issues were addressed in the STAR*D study (Rush et al., 2004). This study involved 1,439 patients with major depression, all of whom did not attain a satisfactory response to the Level 1 medication citalopram, a selective serotonin reuptake inhibitor (SSRI). These patients were randomized to Level 2 treatments, which included four possible switch options (i.e., sertraline, bupropion, venlafaxine, cognitive therapy) and three citalopram augmentation options (i.e., bupropion, buspirone, cognitive therapy; see Figure 7.1). Patients who still did not demonstrate an adequate response to their Level 2 treatment were eligible for random assignment at Level 3 to two switch options (i.e., mirtazapine or nortriptyline) and to two augment options (i.e., lithium or thyroid hormone). Those who still failed to achieve adequate response could be randomized to one of two Level 4 switch options. The goal of the study was to determine the best treatment option for patients at each level.

The STAR*D study represented a combination of the two approaches to designing the adaptive studies described earlier. A panel of depression treatment experts and researchers worked out the possible treatment options at each of the four levels through a consensus process, making use of existing data and clinical experience. The study then used experimental procedures to determine the best treatment option at each level for patients who failed to respond at the prior level. In addition, the study is an excellent example of a sequential randomization paradigm (Murphy et al., 2007) in which patients can be randomized multiple times. One important issue not addressed by the STAR*D design is what to do with responders. Should such patients be continued on their current medication, and if so, for how long?

One of the more interesting features of this study was that patients were randomized only within the treatment conditions that they were willing to

Step 1: All participants given trial of citalopram.

Step 2: Nonresponders to Step 1 (*n* =1,439) randomized[a] to

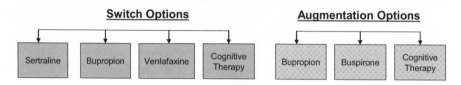

Step 3: Nonresponders to Step 2 rerandomized[a] to

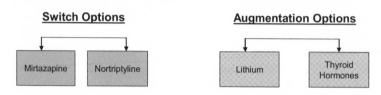

Figure 7.1. Sequenced Treatment Alternatives to Relieve Depression (STAR*D) study design. Data from Rush et al. (2004).
[a]Patients randomized only to those conditions they would actually accept.

accept. This design feature was included to address a common problem in clinical trials—that is, patients end up randomized to a treatment they do not want, and therefore they either never receive the treatment or receive a clearly inadequate dose. The large sample size of the study made such a design feasible. As it turned out, the possible comparisons between the seven Level 2 options were limited by the large numbers of patients who ended up selecting only a limited number of conditions to which they could be randomized. For example, of the 1,439 nonresponding patients who enrolled in Level 2, only 21 were willing to be randomized to all of the seven conditions. Furthermore, only 147 patients were willing to be randomized to a condition that included cognitive therapy (Rush et al., 2006). Because of strong patient preference, the investigators had to look separately at patients who were only willing to be randomized to various switch options (*n* = 727) and those only willing to be randomized to augmentation options (*n* = 565).

Results for the switch arm at Level 2 indicated no difference in depression outcomes, tolerability, or adverse events between the three medication conditions (Rush et al., 2006). However, one in four patients who were nonresponders at Level 1 had a remission of symptoms after switching to a different antidepressant at Level 2. In the augmentation arm, some group differences were observed. Patients who received bupropion in addition to citalopram had a greater reduction in the number and severity of symptoms, fewer side effects, and fewer adverse events than those whose treatment was augmented with buspirone. There were no differences in rates of remission from depression, however (approximately 30%; Trivedi et al., 2006). The outcomes in these two arms could not be directly compared because most participants had self-selected into one of the two arms at the time of randomization.

Analyses from the Level 3 switch arm of the study indicated that remission rates for patients who had failed to achieve remission in Levels 1 and 2 were only approximately 15% and did not differ across the two conditions (i.e., mirtazapine vs. nortriptyline; Fava et al., 2006). Data from the augmentation arm also did not find differences in depression outcomes between the two options (i.e., lithium vs. triiodothyronine), although triiodothyronine produced fewer side effects and was better tolerated than lithium (Niernberg et al., 2006). Remission rates were approximately 20% in this arm.

Therefore, in the end, STAR*D did not yield algorithms that provided specific guidance on what to do next with nonresponders to citalopram. Rather, the main conclusion of the study was that treatment providers should continue to try various switches or augmentations because each successive modification in medication generated additional responders. In addition, patient preference and medication side effect profiles turned out to be important factors to consider when selecting treatment approaches for initial nonresponders.

Treatment for Hypertension

Another large-scale medication study that followed an adaptive model was the Antihypertensive and Lipid-Lowering Treatment to Prevent Heart Attack Trial (ALLHAT; ALLHAT Collaborative Research Group, 2002). This trial randomized more than 33,000 participants to one of three medication conditions: a diuretic (i.e., chlorthalidone), a calcium channel blocker (CCB; i.e., amlodipine), or an ACE inhibitor (i.e., lisinopril). Patients were monitored quarterly in the 1st year and every 4 months after that up to 8 years. The goal was to achieve good blood pressure control as indicated by readings of less than 140/90 mm Hg.

The adaptive component of the protocol indicated that when patients failed to achieve the blood pressure goal, physicians were to increase the dose of the assigned study drug and add additional medications (i.e., Step 2 or Step 3 medications) when necessary. Three medications were recommended as Step 2 drugs, with physicians instructed to choose the one they thought would be most effective. One additional medication was selected as a Step 3 drug, for those who failed to respond to the Step 2 augmentation. This study was adaptive in that it involved the close monitoring of a tailoring variable—blood pressure—and clear guidance on when to make a change to the initial treatment routine. However, the protocol did not dictate which medication to select for augmentation if adequate blood pressure control was not achieved.

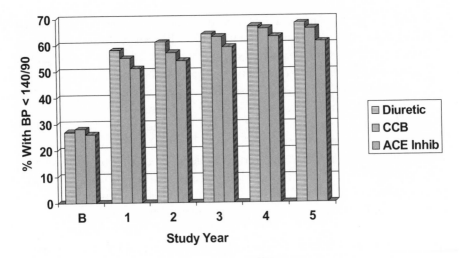

Figure 7.2. Blood pressure results in the Antihypertensive and Lipid-Lowering Treatment to Prevent Heart Attack Trial. Data from ALLHAT Collaborative Research Group (2002). BP = blood pressure; B = baseline; CCB = calcium channel blocker; ACE Inhib = angiotensin-converting enzyme inhibitor.

At the end of the 1st year of the study, less than 30% of the study participants had achieved the blood pressure goal of less than 140/90 mm Hg (see Figure 7.2). However, by Year 5, more than 60% had achieved this goal. As can be seen in Figure 7.3, these improvements may have been related to the increased use of medication augmentation as the study progressed. Rates of augmentation with Step 2 or 3 medication rose from under 30% in Year 1 to more than 40% in Year 5.

Providing Feedback to Therapists Treating Behavioral Disorders

Psychotherapy researchers have focused considerably more attention than addiction researchers on what happens between therapist and patient within a psychotherapy session and how that is related to changes in symptoms over the following week or at later points (Orlinsky, Ronnestad, & Willutzki, 2004). These data are obtained in several ways. The gold standard involves audio- or videotaping entire sessions and applying coding systems to rate the behavior and statements of both patient and therapist. Data have also been obtained through brief questionnaires completed by patients and therapists after the session. Information on changes in symptoms (e.g., depression scores) is then obtained at the beginning of the next therapy session and at subsequent points. This assessment paradigm can also be used to adjust the content or intensity of treatment. Specifically, data collected regularly from patients are used to modify subsequent treatment for those who are not demonstrating an adequate treatment response (Howard, Moras, Brill,

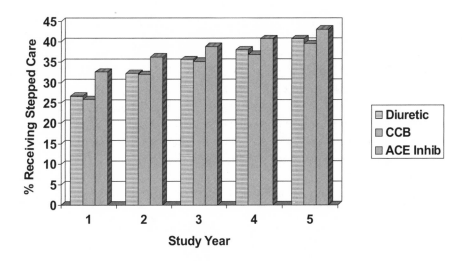

Figure 7.3. Use of Step 2 or 3 medication augmentation in Antihypertensive and Lipid-Lowering Treatment to Prevent Heart Attack Trial. Data from ALLHAT Collaborative Research Group (2002). CCB = calcium channel blocker; ACE Inhib = angiotensin-converting enzyme inhibitor.

Martinovich, & Lutz, 1996; Lambert, Hansen, & Finch, 2001; Lueger et al., 2001).

In a study by Lambert, Whipple, et al. (2001), 609 patients being treated by 31 therapists in a university counseling center were randomized to feedback or no feedback conditions. Data on changes in symptoms during the course of treatment were obtained using a short questionnaire administered at the beginning of each session. During the study, therapists in the feedback condition were given information each week on whether the patient was in one of four possible categories: now functioning in the normal range, experiencing adequate improvement, experiencing less than adequate improvement, or in danger of imminent dropout. In the patients who were considered to not be progressing as expected ($n = 66$), the provision of feedback to the therapists was associated with better retention and outcomes than no feedback. In the patients who were progressing as expected ($n = 543$), feedback did not further improve outcomes but did reduce the number of sessions provided.

It should be noted that in the Lambert, Whipple, et al. (2001) study, the adaptive protocol included a tailoring variable with specified cutting points and decision rules stating that therapists were supposed to modify their approach if patients got certain scores on that measure. However, the adaptive protocol did not provide explicit guidelines for what the therapists should do differently when faced with poor patient response, as was also the case in the ALLHAT study. The selection of potential modifications was simply left up to the therapists. This raises an interesting question about the potential value of more explicit algorithms that are designed, in a sense, to override clinical judgment regarding modifications to treatment. Do clinicians need to be given a blueprint for how to conduct treatment, or is the availability of standardized data on whether patients are progressing reasonably well sufficient to improve practice? The answer to these questions may depend on a number of factors, including the range of potential treatment options for nonresponders, the strength of the evidence base regarding the effectiveness of those options, and level of training, and experience of the clinician.

Computerized Tailoring of Smoking Cessation Messages

A recent study by Strecher et al. (2005) provided an interesting example of the use of computerized algorithms to generate adaptive interventions. In this study, callers to a cancer information service were randomized to receive one of four interventions after a baseline assessment interview: a single, untailored smoking cessation guide (SU); a single, tailored smoking cessation guide (ST); a series of four printed materials tailored to the baseline assessment only (MT); or a series of four printed materials tailored to baseline and then retailored using data from a 5-month progress assessment (MRT). All intervention materials were delivered through the mail. The tailoring made use of information on a wide range of factors, including motives for quitting, previous quit attempts, barriers to quitting, social support, smoking status of social supports, age, and gender. In the MRT group, data on stage of change, motives, barriers, and social support were updated at the 5-month point, and materials received thereafter were modified on the basis of these new data.

At the 12-month follow-up, there was no difference in 7-day point prevalence smoking abstinence rates between the four conditions. However, the two multiple message groups (MT and MRT) had higher quit rates than the two single message groups. Analyses were also done on the subsample of participants who reported that they were not smoking at the 5-month point. In this group, those receiving the multiple retailored messages (MRT) had higher quit rates at 12 months than those in the other three conditions. Shifting the focus of the material to help specifically with relapse prevention appeared to have a beneficial effect in those participants who had managed to stop smoking by Month 5.

CONCLUSION

Tailoring treatments solely on the basis of information collected at intake may be of limited value, at least in the case of chronic disorders in which symptoms and status are expected to wax and wane over time. Adaptive treatment—the regular monitoring of progress over time and use of decision rules to change treatment when necessary—holds real promise as a means to better manage chronic disorders. However, there is a potential catch. One of the core assumptions of adaptive treatment is that patients who are not responding adequately to one intervention will respond to a different intervention. In many diseases and disorders, there is evidence to support this assumption (e.g., hypertension, depression, infection, cancer). STAR*D, for example, showed that even if careful research could not identify the best switch or augment option for a patient who did not respond to an initial SSRI, it made sense to keep switching or augmenting medications until response was achieved.

In the case of patients with substance use disorders, however, it is not clear that this core assumption of adaptive treatment can really be met. After all, patients with substance use disorders often communicate their lack of a good treatment response by dropping out, which of course makes it difficult to switch or augment their treatment protocol. However, as research described in chapter 8 clearly illustrates, effective adaptive protocols have been developed for substance use disorders. These studies have directly addressed the tendency of nonresponders to drop out of treatment by including features such as incentives, aggressive outreach, motivational interviewing, and telephone contact in the interventions. In addition, some studies have used patients' desire to receive a particular treatment, such as methadone, as leverage to increase compliance and accept changes in treatment intensity.

8

ADAPTIVE TREATMENT
IN THE ADDICTIONS

Although research on adaptive approaches to treatment has a relatively short history in most fields, including addiction treatment, a number of such studies have been done with patients who have alcohol or drug use disorders. Most of these studies have tested adaptive protocols put together by expert consensus and patient feedback rather than through experimental means. In this chapter, examples of stepped care, extended adaptive monitoring, and adaptive continuation treatments, and the results generated by these studies, are presented and discussed.

STEPPED CARE

In the stepped-care approach (Breslin et al., 1999; Breslin, Sobell, Sobell, Buchan, & Cunningham, 1997; M. B. Sobell & Sobell, 2000), patients are started at the lowest appropriate level of care, and then "stepped up" to more intensive treatment if warranted by poor initial response. This approach has the potential to increase rates of participation because it may be more palatable to patients given that it places a lower burden on them at the beginning of treatment. Stepped care may also increase cost-effectiveness and cost-benefit, because lower intensity treatments are also often less costly. However, the approach also runs the risk of yielding poorer outcomes if a significant proportion of patients do not do well in the initial treatment or if those who do poorly drop out before receiving an intensification of treatment.

Breslin et al. (1999) evaluated a stepped-care intervention for problem drinkers. Participants who continued to drink during an initial four-session intervention were randomly assigned to receive or not receive an additional counseling session and two supplemental personalized progress reports. The results indicated no differences in drinking outcomes between the two groups, although this was not surprising given the low intensity of the additional treatment and the small sample size.

Bischof et al. (2008) recently reported on the effectiveness of a telephone-based stepped-care approach for individuals identified as problem drinkers in medical practices in Germany. In this study, 408 individuals who screened positive for alcohol use disorders were randomly assigned to receive one of three conditions: usual care, full care, or stepped care. Both the full-care and stepped-care models included a computerized intervention plus up to four subsequent telephone-based intervention sessions. In the stepped-care version, the number of telephone contacts delivered was governed by how well the individual responded to the intervention. In the full-care version, the intervention was fixed at four telephone contacts. Both active interventions produced better drinking outcomes at 12 months compared with standard care. Although participants in the stepped-care condition received roughly half as much treatment as those in the full-care condition, their drinking outcomes were the same. Therefore, the stepped-care algorithm reduced both burden to the participant and cost to the system, with no compromise on effectiveness.

Brooner and Kidorf (2002) developed a stepped-care treatment for methadone patients that features three levels of counseling intensity. Patients begin in Step 1, which consists of one individual counseling session and one group educational session per week. If patients miss a counseling session or have a drug-positive urine test, they are moved to Step 2, which includes a second weekly group session. Further missed sessions or drug-positive urine tests result in transfer to Step 3, which involves two individual and five group sessions per week. Patients who have been stepped up can move back down to Step 1 by attending all counseling sessions and providing drug-free urine samples. Studies by this group indicate that this stepped-care approach works equally well in methadone clinics or at physicians' offices (King et al., 2002) and can be adapted to increase employment rates in methadone patients (Kidorf, Neufeld, & Brooner, 2004).

As has been noted in this book, one of the challenges to the successful implementation of adaptive protocols is low rates of compliance with increases in level of care. Brooner et al. (2004) tested whether the incorporation of additional contingencies to motivate adherence would improve the performance of their stepped-care protocol. These contingencies were less convenient methadone dosing times and methadone taper coupled with possible discharge, which were implemented as a consequence of missed counseling sessions. Compared with standard stepped care alone, the combination of behavioral contingencies plus stepped care produced a higher rate of counseling attendance (83% vs. 44% of session attended) and a lower rate of poor treatment response (46% vs. 79%).

Recently, Brooner et al. (2007) directly compared their adaptive stepped-care approach with a contingency management (CM) approach in 236 treatment-seeking opioid-dependent patients entering a methadone clinic. The study condition that provided both stepped care and CM produced the highest rate of drug-negative urine samples over the 9-month study period (60% in Months 1–6; 53% in Months 7–9). The stepped-care and CM-only conditions were not different from each other on this outcome (approximately 48% negative in both time periods), but both were better than standard care at the methadone clinic (29% negative in Months 1–6; 33% in Months 7–9). With regard to participation in treatment, the stepped-care protocol produced better adherence to scheduled counseling sessions, whereas the CM condition produced better overall retention.

Another approach to stepped care for opiate dependence was developed and recently evaluated by Kakko et al. (2007). Methadone has proved effectiveness in treating opiate dependence, but there are some concerns about its safety and whether the clinics at which it is dispensed are optimal recovery environments. A newer medication, buprenorphine, has several potential advantages over methadone; it has a better safety profile and can be dispensed in office-based practices rather than in drug treatment clinics. However, it may not be as effective as methadone, at least not for all opiate addicts. This suggests a potential adaptive treatment strategy for opioid dependence in which individuals are started on buprenorphine and then switched to methadone if they do not have a sufficiently positive response.

To test the effectiveness of such an approach, Kakko et al. (2007) compared two approaches to opiate dependence treatment: a fixed treatment that starts patients directly on methadone maintenance versus a stepped-care algorithm that begins with buprenorphine and escalates to methadone only if warranted by poor response. The results of the study indicated that the two treatment conditions yielded similar results with regard to retention (78% retained at 6 months), opiate use, other drug use, and other addiction-related problem severity as measured by the Addiction Severity Index. Among completers in the stepped-care group, 54% were switched from buprenorphine to methadone. Therefore, the advantage of the stepped-care algorithm was that it reduced patient burden and increased safety, without sacrificing good substance use outcomes. It is interesting to note that age, sex, duration of heroin use, or baseline problem severity did not predict which patients in the stepped-care condition were switched to methadone. This lack of moderation effects points out that often progress in treatment, rather than baseline severity, is the best indicator of need to adapt or modify treatment.

Marlowe et al. (2008) recently conducted a pilot study of an adaptive drug court protocol. This new study builds on their earlier work in which risk level assessed at the start of drug court was used to match offenders to optimal hearing schedules. The new study once again assigned offenders to biweekly or as-needed hearing schedules on the basis of risk but then further adapted hearing schedules on the basis of outcomes in drug court. Offenders who were continuing to attend drug court as scheduled but were using drugs were provided with intensive clinical case management to help them address the problems that were contributing to relapse. In contrast, those who failed to attend scheduled drug court sessions were increased to biweekly hearings if they were on the as-needed schedule or were terminated from the program and sentenced on their original drug charges (i.e., likely leading to incarceration) if they were already on the biweekly schedule.

Several results from this pilot study were notable. First, the adaptive algorithm was acceptable to both offenders and staff and was implemented as planned in 85% of the situations in which offenders met criteria for adaptive changes. This strongly suggests that adaptive protocols can achieve good compliance with recommended modifications in care, as long as the right incentives are built in for the participants. Second, the full adaptive algorithm with baseline matching produced better drug use outcomes than standard drug court (e.g., 64% vs. 48% of all urine samples were drug free; 8.9 vs. 6.9 consecutive drug-free urine samples provided). Analyses of mechanisms of action indicated that drug court responded much more rapidly to poor performance on the part of the offenders in the adaptive condition, relative to drug court as usual.

EXTENDED ADAPTIVE MONITORING

Another approach to disease management in the addictions is extended monitoring with an adaptive component. This approach can be considered adaptive because patients can be switched from low-intensity monitoring to more intensive forms of treatment if they are not doing well, according to predetermined decision rules.

One such study was the Foote and Erfurt (1991) employee assistance program continuing care project described in chapter 3. In this protocol, participants received an average of 15 contacts over a 1-year period, including seven visits and three telephone calls. Although the planned schedule of contacts was weekly for 1 month, monthly for the next 5 months, and bimonthly after that, the contact schedule reverted to once per week in the case of relapse or threat of relapse. The experimental condition produced better outcomes than the standard follow-up procedure on substance abuse treatment costs and hospitalizations. However, because substance use outcomes were not assessed in this study, it is not clear whether the adaptive protocol actually reduced alcohol and drug use more than standard care.

Scott, Dennis, and colleagues from Chestnut Health Systems have developed a protocol that they refer to as recovery management checkups (RMC), which is designed to better manage patients with substance use disorders over time (Scott & Dennis 2002). In this protocol, substance abusers who have entered treatment are followed and interviewed every 3 months. For those not currently in treatment or in a controlled environment such as jail, need for further treatment is determined through a relatively brief assessment. The criteria for needing further treatment consists of meeting any of the following over the prior 90 days: use of any substance(s) on 13 or more days; being drunk or high for most of 1 or more days; not meeting work, school, or home responsibilities on 1 or more days; having substance use–related problems in the prior month; having withdrawal symptoms in the prior week; or the desire to return to treatment. Individuals who met criteria for need for treatment are immediately transferred to a linkage manager, who uses motivational interviewing techniques to help the participant recognize and acknowledge the problem and need for treatment, addresses any existing barriers to reentering treatment, and arranges scheduling and transportation to treatment.

The RMC protocol was evaluated in a study in which 448 adults presenting at a central intake unit were randomized to RMC or quarterly research follow-ups and followed for 24 months (Dennis, Scott, & Funk, 2003; Scott, Dennis, & Foss, 2005). The results of the study indicated that the RMC intervention led to better management of the patients over time. First, patients in RMC were more likely to be readmitted to treatment (60% vs. 51%), were readmitted sooner (mean of 376 vs. 600 days), and received more treatment during the 2-year follow-up (mean of 62 vs. 40 days) than those in the control condition. Second, patients in RMC had better substance use outcomes over the course of the follow-up than those in the control condition. Specifically, RMC patients were less likely to meet criteria for needing treatment in five or more quarters than patients in the control condition (23% vs. 32%) and were less likely to be in need of treatment in the final quarter of the follow-up (43% vs. 56%). These effects were generally small but consistently favored RMC over the comparison condition.

The Chestnut Health group conducted a second study with a version of RMC that was modified on the basis of some of the limitations observed in the first study (Scott & Dennis, in press). The self-report assessment used to determine need for treatment was augmented with urine testing, which increased the percentage of participants who were found to need treatment at each assessment point (44% vs. 30% of those interviewed). Transportation assistance was provided to increase the percentage of participants found to be in need of treatment who actually completed an intake assessment. Finally, several practices were put in place to increase retention in those participants who did complete an intake appointment at a treatment program. These practices involved closer collaboration between the research team and the treatment programs to reengage participants in treatment who drop out after intake and to prevent hasty administrative discharges. These modifications increased the effectiveness of the intervention to a considerable degree (Scott & Dennis, in press). For example, higher percentages of participants attended intake assessments (42% vs. 30% of those in need of treatment), completed a treatment intake (30% vs. 25%), and remained in treatment for a minimum of 14 days (58% vs. 39%). Moreover, the improved RMC intervention produced significantly more days of abstinence during the 2-year follow-up (mean of 480 vs. 430, $p < .05$, $d = 0.29$) than the comparison condition, an effect that was not obtained in the first study. However, this effect, which translates into about 2 additional days of abstinence per month, was relatively small in magnitude.

A study conducted in Sweden examined the effect of an extended intervention for middle-aged, heavy-drinking men that consisted of brief visits with a physician every 3 months and monthly visits with a nurse that included a test of gamma glutamyl transferase (GGT) levels (Kristenson, Ohlin, Hulten-Nosslin, Trell, & Hood 1983). GGT is a liver function measure obtained from blood samples that can be used as an indicator of sustained heavy drinking. The intervention lasted for up to 4 years and was compared with standard care, which consisted of an initial screening, feedback on GGT test results by mail, and invitations every 2 years to repeat the GGT test.

The experimental intervention was adapted on the basis of GGT levels in the following manner. Patients who were able to reduce their GGT levels by cutting back significantly on their drinking were given some flexibility in choice of drinking goals (e.g., reduction vs. abstinence). However, if GGT levels were not reduced or were increased, abstinence became the only acceptable goal of treatment. The frequency of therapeutic contact was also reduced after sustained reductions in GGT were achieved. Results indicated that compared with those in the control condition, participants who received the extended monitoring intervention had fewer sick days (80% reduction) and fewer hospital days (60% reduction) over the first 4 years of the follow-up and lower mortality rates (50% reduction) over the full 6-year follow-up. Longer term mortality rates (e.g., 10–16 years) were also lower in the extended intervention condition (10.4% vs. 13.9%, $p = .03$; Kristenson, Osterling, Nilsson, & Lindgarde, 2002).

ADAPTIVE CONTINUATION TREATMENTS

In the addictions, several studies have examined the effectiveness of step-down, or continuing care, models for patients who are initial treatment responders. The American Society of Addiction Medicine (ASAM) attempted to provide guidelines on when patients could be stepped down from more to less intensive interventions through its continuing care criteria (ASAM, 2001). As discussed in chapter 6, the ASAM placement system assesses patients in six problem areas or dimensions. According to the continuing care criteria, patients are to be maintained at the higher level of care until they qualify for a lower level of care on all six dimensions. Although these criteria make intuitive sense, they have not been formally evaluated.

Naltrexone Continuation

O'Malley et al. (2003) conducted a study of naltrexone in alcohol-dependent patients, which focused on optimal continuation treatments for initial responders. Patients were first randomized to either naltrexone plus primary medical care–based counseling or naltrexone plus specialized alcohol counseling, which in this case was cognitive–behavioral therapy (CBT). Patients in each condition who achieved what was considered to be a good response to the medication over a 10-week period (57% of the original sample) were then randomized for a second time to either extended naltrexone or placebo, along with continuation of the behavioral treatment they had been receiving in Phase 1. The continuation treatments were provided for an additional 24 weeks. Because it employed two randomizations, this study can be considered an example of a sequential multiple-assignment randomized trial study (Murphy et al., 2007; see also chap. 7, this volume).

The results indicated that there were essentially no differences between the primary care and CBT conditions on primary drinking outcomes during the first 10-week phase of the study. However, differences were observed in the 24-week continuation phase. Specifically, patients receiving primary care–based counseling had better drinking outcomes if they received extended naltrexone, including greater percentage days abstinent (89.8% vs. 78.4%), fewer drinks per drinking day (mean of 2.1 vs. 3.0), and lower scores on a biological measure of heavy drinking. Moreover, 81% of those in the naltrexone condition were categorized as responders, compared with only 52% in the placebo condition. Conversely, those who received CBT did not benefit from extended naltrexone (O'Malley et al., 2003). This study is a nice illustration of how the effectiveness of later treatment interventions can vary as a function of which intervention patients received earlier in the protocol.

Continuing Care for Completers of Intensive Outpatient Treatment

Our group at the University of Pennsylvania conducted an initial adaptive study with cocaine-dependent patients who had completed a 4-week intensive outpatient program (IOP; McKay et al., 1997, 1999). Participants in this study ($N = 132$) were randomly assigned to two 6-month continuing care interventions: group counseling or individualized relapse prevention. After completing baseline assessments at the beginning of the continuing care phase of treatment, they were followed for 2 years. This study is also described briefly in Table 3.1.

The first intervention was 12-step-oriented group counseling (two sessions/week). The sessions consisted primarily of discussions of urges to use and any relapses, advice and feedback on working the steps of the Alcoholics Anonymous program, guidance on constructive planning of unstructured time, and exhortations to avoid risky situations. This intervention represented standard continuing care in most private or publicly funded treatment clinics.

The second intervention was cognitive–behavioral relapse prevention (RP; Annis & Davis, 1989), provided through one individual and one group session per week. Each individual session was highly structured through a series of modules, which also provided weekly homework assignments. As is the case in most CBT–RP protocols, this intervention used functional analysis to identify personal relapse triggers, helped patients to anticipate when they might encounter their own relapse triggers, and provided help in developing and practicing new coping responses to those risky situations.

Treatment Main Effects

There was little evidence of any differences between the two conditions in cocaine use outcomes over the 2-year follow-up, including percentage days of cocaine use, time to first relapse, monetary value of cocaine used, categorical abstinence measures, or urine toxicology (McKay et al., 1999, 2001). The only differences that did emerge were (a) higher rates of total cocaine abstinence in the first 3 months of the follow-up in patients who received group counseling rather than RP and (b) less severe cocaine relapses among those with any cocaine use who received RP rather than group counseling (McKay et al., 1997). Given the number of comparisons made, these findings could have been due to chance, although they are consistent with the theoretical underpinnings of the total abstinence orientation of the12-step-based group counseling condition and the harm reduction orientation of RP.

Analyses of Adaptive Effects

With regard to adaptive treatment, we focused on progress during IOP as a possible tailoring variable. Specifically, we hypothesized that IOP graduates who had been able to achieve remission from current cocaine dependence during IOP would do well in either continuing care protocol, but we expected treatment group differences to emerge in those patients who continued to meet current dependence criteria because of ongoing cocaine use while in IOP (24% of the sample). Specifically, RP was predicted to be more effective with these patients than group counseling. We based this prediction on the emphasis in RP on (a) teaching patients to be able to recognize their own relapse triggers, (b) developing improved coping responses for those situations, and (c) rehearsing the new coping responses. In addition, the fact that RP in this study included individual treatment sessions, and thereby greater individualized attention, was considered important with patients who had not been able to stop using cocaine in a group-based intervention.

The results closely mirrored what had been predicted. Patients who had achieved remission from current cocaine dependence had excellent outcomes in both continuing care conditions, with average frequency of cocaine use remaining at approximately 5% for the entire 24-month follow-up. Patients who had not been able to achieve remission from cocaine dependence and were randomly assigned to group counseling continuing care averaged 16% days of cocaine use throughout the follow-up. However, the nonremitted patients who received RP used cocaine on only 6% of the days in Months 1 through 6 and averaged 10% days cocaine use for the remainder of the follow-up. Therefore, RP was particularly effective, especially for the first 6 months, in these patients who had failed to achieve remission from cocaine dependence before entering continuing care.

Approximately 86% of the patients in the study carried a lifetime diagnosis of alcohol dependence, in addition to cocaine dependence. Moreover, about 16% of the sample still met criteria for current alcohol dependence at the end of IOP. Therefore, we also examined whether remission from alcohol dependence during IOP might also be a good tailoring variable in an algorithm to place patients in optimal continuing care following IOP. As had been the case with cocaine dependence and cocaine outcomes, a significant interaction between current alcohol dependence status at the end of IOP and alcohol use outcomes over the 24 months was obtained. This time, however, the treatment effect favoring RP over group counseling in patients who had not achieved remission from alcohol dependence was found in Year 2 of the follow-up, rather than in the first 6 months. Therefore, there was a sleeper effect, similar to effects reported by Carroll and others for CBT (Carroll et al., 1994).

Telephone Continuing Care Following Intensive Outpatient Programs

After the completion of this first adaptive study, our group conducted a second randomized continuing care study with initial responders to IOP. This second study, which was also described briefly in chapter 3, featured three continuing care interventions, each of which was provided for 12 weeks after discharge from IOP. These interventions were two conditions from the prior study, group counseling, and RP, plus a third condition that involved telephone-based continuing care (TEL). The patients in the study (N = 359) had all completed 4-week long IOPs and had provided at least one drug-free

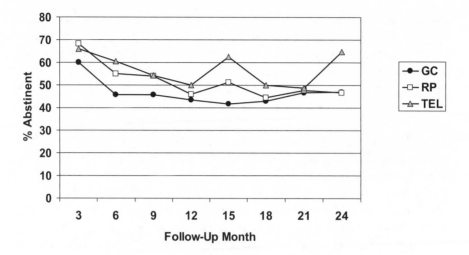

Figure 8.1. Total abstinence rates in each 3-month segment of follow-up. TEL > Group Counseling, *p* < .05. GC = group counseling; RP = relapse prevention; TEL = telephone-based continuing care. From "The Effectiveness of Telephone Based Continuing Care for Alcohol and Cocaine Dependence: 24-Month Outcomes," by J. R. McKay, K. G. Lynch, D. S. Shepard, and H. M. Pettinati, 2005, *Archives of General Psychiatry, 62*, p. 204. Copyright © 2005, American Medical Association. All rights reserved. Adapted with permission.

urine sample in the final week of IOP. Half the sample had current dependence on both alcohol and cocaine when they entered the IOP, 25% were dependent on alcohol only, and 25% were dependent on cocaine only. Once again, patients were followed for 2 years following entrance into continuing care (McKay, Lynch, et al., 2004).

The new intervention in this study was a multimodal protocol based primarily on telephone contacts. Each patient in this condition received an initial individual face-to-face orientation session, which was used to introduce the patient to the protocol, go over administrative matters such as safety contracts and alternative contacts, and provide a self-monitoring workbook to be completed before each call. Most important, this session also helped to facilitate an initial connection between the counselor and patient. The patient then received counseling via weekly telephone contacts. These calls were typically 15 to 20 minutes in length and focused on solving one or two problems that were present at that point.

The calls began with a review of the self-monitoring data on substance use and self-help participation from the current week and a review of progress toward the specific goals that had been established for that week. The last portion of the calls was reserved for the development of coping responses for a current or anticipated stressor or risky situation. Patients in this condition were also eligible to attend a loosely structured support group for the first 4

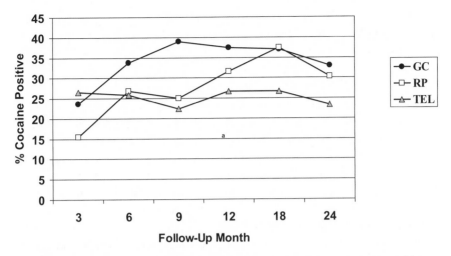

Figure 8.2. Cocaine urine toxicology at each follow-up. Rates of cocaine-positive urines increased more rapidly in RP versus TEL (*p* = .03) and in GC versus TEL (*p* = .05). GC = group counseling; RP = relapse prevention; TEL = telephone-based continuing care. From "The Effectiveness of Telephone Based Continuing Care for Alcohol and Cocaine Dependence: 24-Month Outcomes," by J. R. McKay, K. G. Lynch, D. S. Shepard, and H. M. Pettinati, 2005, *Archives of General Psychiatry*, *62*, p. 204. Copyright © 2005, American Medical Association. All rights reserved. Adapted with permission.

weeks of the protocol (1 session/week), to help them transition from 9 hours of treatment per week in IOP down to a 15- to 20-minute telephone call.

Treatment Main Effects

In analyses of main effects, outcomes in the telephone condition were surprisingly good and consistently better than those in RP and group counseling. The study had two primary self-report substance use outcome measures: total abstinence from alcohol and cocaine within each 3-month segment of the follow-up (yes–no) and percentage days abstinent within each segment. The TEL condition produced significantly higher rates of abstinence than group counseling within the 3-month segments over the 2-year follow-up (average of approximately 65% vs. 50% across the 3-month segments; see Figure 8.1). Abstinence outcomes in RP were between those in TEL and group counseling and not significantly different from either.

In alcohol-dependent patients, TEL produced significantly better improvements than RP from baseline to 24 months on a biological indicator of drinking, the liver function measure GGT. Scores on other liver function measures and percentage days heavy drinking at 12 months also indicated an advantage to TEL over group counseling and RP. In cocaine-dependent patients, a Group × Time interaction was observed with cocaine urine toxicology tests obtained at each follow-up. In this interaction, the advantage of TEL over RP and group counseling increased over the course of the 2-year follow-up (TEL vs. RP, p = .03; TEL vs. Group Counseling, p = .05; see Figure 8.2; see also McKay, Lynch, et al., 2004; McKay, Lynch, Shepard, & Pettinati, 2005).

Analyses of Adaptive Effects

With regard to adaptive treatment algorithms, analyses were performed to determine whether progress toward key therapeutic goals of IOP could be used to identify which patients would do best in each of the three continuing care conditions. The measures of progress that were examined were alcohol use in IOP, drug use in IOP, current psychiatric symptom severity, self-help involvement, general social support from family and friends, commitment to abstinence, readiness to change, and self-efficacy. The measures were selected on the basis of discussions with IOP directors and clinicians to identify key goals in the IOP phase of treatment, as well as reviews of the clinical literature on IOP. In addition, these variables had all been significant predictors of outcome in a number of prior studies, as describe in chapter 2. Potential matching effects between two other variables assessed at entrance to IOP, number of current substance dependence diagnoses and lifetime depression diagnosis, and performance within each continuing care condition were also examined.

The results of the analyses indicated that no one measure was a good predictor of differential outcomes within each condition (see chap. 10 for more details about these analyses). However, a composite risk indicator scale made up of the sum of dichotomized scores from seven measures did interact significantly with treatment condition to predict abstinence outcomes. The seven measures in the scale were as follows: any alcohol use in IOP, any cocaine use in IOP, lack of commitment to total abstinence at the end of IOP, low self-help participation during IOP, low social support during IOP, low self-efficacy at end of IOP, and current dependence at intake to IOP on both alcohol and cocaine. Scores on the risk indicator measure ranged from 0 to 7 (mean = 2.5), with higher scores indicating poorer progress in IOP and co-occurring alcohol and cocaine dependence (see Figure 8.3). Although all the patients in the study sample could be considered responders because they were able to complete IOP and achieve abstinence in at least the last week of IOP, these data indicated a fair degree of variability in progress toward key therapeutic goals during IOP.

Overall, higher scores on the risk indicator predicted a lower likelihood of abstinence in each of the 3-month quarters of the 2-year follow-up. However, as indicated in the four panels of Figure 8.4, the slope of that effect was steeper in the TEL condition than in either RP or group counseling. Patients with risk indicator scores of 3 or lower typically had better outcomes in TEL as opposed to RP or group counseling, whereas those with scores of 4 or greater did better in group counseling than in TEL. This effect was found in each quarter of the follow-up through Month 21 (McKay, Lynch, Shepard,

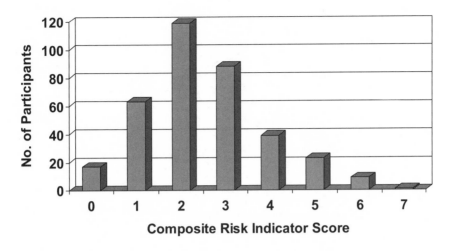

Figure 8.3. Distribution of scores on the composite risk indicator. Mean score = 2.50.

Morgenstern, et al., 2005; McKay, Lynch, Shepard, & Pettinati, 2005). The main effect favoring TEL over group counseling was accounted for by the fact that only approximately 20% of the study sample had a risk indicator score of 4 or higher.

The results of these analyses suggest that patients with current dependence on only one substance who make at least moderately good progress toward the goals of IOP will do better in a more flexible, lower intensity continuing care model than in more intensive treatment that requires frequent continued visits to the clinic. Conversely, higher risk patients—those with co-occurring alcohol and cocaine dependence who do not achieve a majority of the central goals of IOP—do not appear ready to step all the way down from IOP to TEL. Rather, they will do better if they receive further face-to-face treatment at the clinic.

CONCLUSION

Although adaptive treatment studies are a relatively new development in addiction treatment research, 15 such studies were identified and reviewed in this chapter. These studies included eight stepped-care studies, four extended adaptive monitoring studies, and three adaptive continuation studies. All but one of these studies (i.e., Breslin et al., 1999) yielded significant results in which adaptive procedures led to either better substance use outcomes or to equivalent outcomes in treatments with other advantages (e.g., lower cost, lower patients burden, greater safety) or produced algorithms that specified which patients would benefit most from what continuation treat-

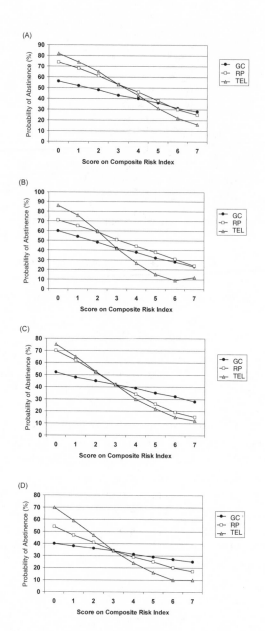

Figure 8.4. Probability of abstinence Months (A) 4 to 6, (B) 7 to 9, (C) 10 to 12, and (D) 13 to 15. (A), (B), and (C) are from "Do Patient Characteristics and Initial Progress in Treatment Moderate the Effectiveness of Telephone-Based Continuing Care for Substance Use Disorders?" by J. R. McKay, K. G. Lynch, D. S. Shepard, J. Morgenstern, R. F Forman, and H. M. Pettinati, 2005, *Addiction, 100*, p. 222. Copyright 2005 by Blackwell. Adapted with permission. (D) is from "The Effectiveness of Telephone Based Continuing Care for Alcohol and Cocaine Dependence: 24-Month Outcomes," by J. R. McKay, K. G. Lynch, D. S. Shepard, and H. M. Pettinati, 2005, *Archives of General Psychiatry, 62*, p. 204. Copyright © 2005, American Medical Association. All rights reserved. Adapted with permission. GC = group counseling; RP = relapse prevention; TEL = telephone-based continuing care.

ments. These results are highly encouraging with regard to the potential acceptability and effectiveness of adaptive interventions for substance use disorders.

It is also worth noting that both approaches to developing adaptive algorithms discussed in chapter 7, the expert consensus and experimental approaches, were represented in the studies reviewed in this chapter. For example, studies by Bischof et al. (2008); Brooner, Kidorf, and colleagues (Brooner et al., 2004, 2007; Kidorf et al., 2004); Dennis et al. (2002); Kakko et al. (2007); and Marlowe et al. (2008) were examples of adaptive protocols developed via expert consensus and reviews of the literature. Conversely, studies by O'Malley et al. (2003) and our group at the University of Pennsylvania (McKay et al., 1999; McKay, McKay, Lynch, & Pettinati, 2005) made use of progress in the initial phase of treatment and randomization to determine the best continuing care intervention for each study participant. In chapter 9, we take a more detailed look at three adaptive continuing care studies that are currently underway at the University of Pennsylvania.

IV

DEVELOPING AND IMPROVING ADAPTIVE CONTINUING CARE INTERVENTIONS

9

A DETAILED LOOK AT CURRENT ADAPTIVE TREATMENT STUDIES

This chapter takes a detailed look at several current studies at the University of Pennsylvania that are developing or evaluating adaptive disease management algorithms in the addictions. The first study makes use of experimental procedures to develop optimal clinical algorithms for alcohol-dependent patients being treated with naltrexone. It is one of the first examples in addiction treatment research of a sequential multiple-assignment randomized trial (SMART; Murphy et al., 2007), as described in chapter 7. The second study tests two extended telephone-based continuing care (TEL) interventions, one of which includes an adaptive stepped-care algorithm. Once again, the participants in this study are alcohol dependent. The third study also evaluates extended TEL, this time for cocaine-dependent patients. Two adaptive interventions are included in the third study, one of which includes incentives for completing telephone sessions and, when in-person stepped-care sessions are recommended, for providing cocaine-free urine samples. These latter two studies are examples of the expert consensus approach to developing adaptive interventions.

ADAPTIVE ALGORITHM FOR
PHARMACOTHERAPY OF ALCOHOLISM

David Oslin and colleagues at the University of Pennsylvania are conducting a study designed to identify optimal treatment approaches for patients who are started on naltrexone (see Zaharakis et al., 2008). Although this medication has consistently shown evidence of efficacy across many clinical trials (O'Brien & McKay, 2007), the magnitude of the effect has tended to be modest. More important, a significant number of individuals are apparently not helped by the medication. Therefore, there is a need to determine optimal treatment regimes for patients who benefit from the medication and for those who do not. Oslin and his collaborators theorized that there were two main reasons why naltrexone might not be effective with certain individuals. First, it works by blocking opiate receptors, which are involved in generating the pleasurable, or rewarding, feelings produced by alcohol, at least in a significant percentage of drinkers. This would explain the positive effect of naltrexone. However, individuals in whom the pleasurable effects of alcohol were mediated through a different pathway might not receive much benefit from this medication (the possible influence of genetics on naltrexone response is discussed in chap. 6, this volume).

Second, many individuals with substance use disorders have a wide range of co-occurring problems that might include other psychiatric disorders such as depression or anxiety, impulse control problems, severe family or social conflict, lack of positive social support for recovery, or a relative paucity of natural reinforcers that might provide strong incentives for recovery. Moreover, many addicted individuals lack basic social skills needed to manage potential relapse situations. Therefore, it was also possible that the effects of naltrexone might be overwhelmed by co-occurring problems, stressors, or lack of good skills to manage high-risk situations.

In this study, Oslin chose to focus not on patients in traditional, or specialty care, addiction treatment programs but on patients who were being seen in a primary care practice–type setting. This decision was made because many individuals with alcohol use disorders do not want treatment in standard addiction programs for a number of reasons, including stigma, employment or family responsibilities, lack of interest in abstinence-oriented treatment, discomfort with group therapy, and so forth (see chap. 1). However, some of these individuals might be willing to accept help for alcohol problems if it could be delivered in another setting (such as a doctor's office), involve minimal behavioral treatment, and permit goals other than total abstinence. Therefore, the purpose of the study was to develop adaptive algorithms for patients receiving pharmacological treatment for alcoholism in primary care.

Study Design and Interventions

All participants in this study started in a treatment protocol referred to as *alcoholism care management*. It consists of brief weekly visits with a nurse, who provides the behavioral components of the treatment as well as the naltrexone (100 mg/day). The behavioral treatment is similar to a protocol developed at the University of Pennsylvania, referred to as *medical management* (Pettinati et al., 2004), that was used in the COMBINE study (Anton et al., 2006). In the initial visit, the nurse reviews the patient's alcohol dependence diagnosis and discusses the negative consequences of drinking. The importance of abstinence is stressed, education about naltrexone is provided, and a medication adherence plan is developed in collaboration with the patient. Attendance at mutual-help programs is recommended. In subsequent visits, the nurse reviews any episodes of drinking, overall functioning, medication adherence, and adverse consequences. Brief counseling and encouragement are provided to those patients who have slips or relapses.

In this study, the initial phase of treatment could continue for up to 8 weeks. If the patient gets through this period with little or no heavy drinking, he or she is placed in the responder arm of the study, which is described subsequently. Patients who experience heavy drinking are placed in the nonresponder arm at the point at which their heavy drinking occurred and randomized to one of two continuing care options. These options are either to switch treatment from naltrexone to a more intensive and multicomponent behavioral intervention or to augment treatment by having the participant remain on naltrexone and also receive the enhanced behavioral intervention. The rationale for these options was that if naltrexone failed because of biological factors in the alcohol reward system, then there would be no benefit for staying on naltrexone when treatment was stepped up. However, if the problem was that the naltrexone signal was being overwhelmed by co-occurring problems, then there would be some benefit to staying on the medication if the other problems could be more successfully addressed through a comprehensive behavioral intervention.

The stepped-care behavioral intervention used in this study was the Combined Behavioral Intervention (CBI), which was also developed for the COMBINE study (Anton et al., 2006). This intervention integrates aspects of cognitive–behavioral therapy (CBT), motivational interviewing (MI), and 12-step facilitation and strives to engage the patient's external support systems. In the first half of the protocol, the patient and counselor work through a set sequence of treatment modules that incorporate MI and CBT components. Later, the patient and counselor can select from a menu of modules, depending on the particular needs of the patient. During all sessions, the counselor uses the MI style. Miller and Rollnick (2002) defined *MI* as a directive method for enhancing the patient's intrinsic motivation to change by exploring and resolving ambivalence. They indicated four key principles: expressing empathy, developing discrepancy, rolling with resistance, and supporting self-efficacy. MI is characterized less by techniques than by "spirit," which is operationalized in terms of collaboration with the patient; evocation of the patient's own perceptions, goals, and values; and respect for the patient's autonomy. This definition allows for great flexibility in clinical application and adaptation. CBI was provided in one hour-long session per week.

Determining Nonresponse to Naltrexone

One of the questions Oslin and colleagues (see Zaharakis et al., 2009) grappled with in designing this study was how much drinking should be required before a participant was declared a nonresponder to naltrexone. Prior research had indicated that naltrexone had a stronger effect on reducing the frequency of *heavy drinking days* (defined as five or more drinks/day in men, four or more in women) than on reducing the frequency of days on which any alcohol was consumed. This makes sense, given that the medication appears to reduce the euphoric or pleasurable feelings that go along with alcohol use. Such a mechanism of action would be expected to limit heavy drinking but not necessarily lead to abstinence. For example, an alcoholic who was taking naltrexone might have something to drink one evening but not experience much in the way of pleasure or euphoria from it. This might lead to less drinking on future occasions because of the reduced reinforcing effect. Drinking might continue at a low level, however, because naltrexone does not make drinking aversive, as does Antabuse.

All this suggested that the criteria for being a naltrexone responder should permit some degree of experimentation with regard to drinking, but the question was, How much? Unfortunately, there was no research literature on which to base such criteria. Therefore, Oslin and colleagues decided to manipulate this variable experimentally. Half the participants in the study were randomized to one condition in which more than 1 heavy drinking day in the 8-week open-label phase of the study placed them in the nonresponder category, whereas the other half were randomized to a condition in which they were not categorized as nonresponders until they had had 5 heavy drinking days.

Responder Arm

Patients whose drinking during the open-label, first phase of the study never reached the threshold for nonresponse (whether 2 or 5 heavy drinking days) were entered into the responder arm of the study. This arm addressed the question of what the best type of continuing care treatment to provide to such patients would be. Because this group of patients had a good initial response to naltrexone, it seemed clear that they should be provided prescriptions to obtain more of the medication. Oslin and colleagues (see Zaharakis et al., 2009) wondered whether also providing regular telephone contact to monitor medication use and address problems as they emerged might improve outcomes, compared with medication only. However, because these patients had done well with a relatively low-intensity psychosocial intervention, it was possible that they would do well with medication only. Therefore, patients in the responder arm were randomly assigned to medication prescriptions only versus prescriptions plus regular telephone calls for 20 weeks.

Comparison of Eight Treatment Algorithms

The Oslin et al. study (see Zaharakis et al., 2009) can be seen as a test of eight adaptive algorithms for alcohol-dependent patients seen through primary care (see Table 9.1). The eight algorithms are formed by crossing the two criteria for nonresponse (i.e., 2 vs. 5 heavy drinking days in the first 8 weeks) and the randomizations into two conditions within both the nonresponder and responder groups. Two of these algorithms are as follows:

1. If patient has more than 1 heavy drinking day, declare as a nonresponder and augment naltrexone and medication management with CBI. If patient is a responder after 8 weeks, provide prescription for continued naltrexone but do not provide telephone disease management. (Algorithm 1 in Table 9.1)
2. If patient has more than 4 heavy drinking days, declare as a nonresponder, add CBT, and discontinue naltrexone. If patient is a responder after 8 weeks, provide prescription for continued naltrexone and add telephone disease management. (Algorithm 8 in Table 9.1)

The Oslin study was not powered to support comparisons between any two of these eight algorithms, because the total planned enrollment was 300 patients. However, there is sufficient power for several a priori designated, focused comparisons between algorithms and for comparisons between larger groups (e.g., the four algorithms based on the "2 heavy drinking days" definition of *nonresponse* vs. the other four algorithms that use the "5 heavy drinking days" definition).

Preliminary Study Outcomes

The final study sample consisted of 302 patients. Of the 151 patients assigned to the "2 heavy drinking days" definition of *nonresponse*, 43 met this criteria for nonresponse. Conversely, of the 151 randomized to the "5 heavy drinking days" definition of nonresponse, only 24 met this second criteria for nonresponse. Therefore, almost twice as many patients were referred to stepped

TABLE 9.1
Adaptive Intervention Strategies Embedded in Oslin Trial

Adaptive intervention	Definition of *nonresponder*	Decision rules for responders	Decision rules for nonresponders
1	> 1 heavy drinking day	Stay with NTX alone	Add CBI to NTX
2	> 1 heavy drinking day	Stay with NTX alone	Switch to CBI alone
3	> 1 heavy drinking day	Add TDM to NTX	Add CBI to NTX
4	> 1 heavy drinking day	Add TDM to NTX	Switch to CBI alone
5	> 4 heavy drinking days	Stay with NTX alone	Add CBI to NTX
6	> 4 heavy drinking days	Stay with NTX alone	Switch to CBI alone
7	> 4 heavy drinking days	Add TDM to NTX	Add CBI to NTX
8	> 4 heavy drinking days	Add TDM to NTX	Switch to CBI alone

Note. NTX = naltrexone; CBI = combine behavioral intervention; TDM = telephone disease management.

care in the group that required less heavy drinking in the criteria for nonresponse. The 183 patients who did not meet their definition of *nonresponse* during Phase 1 were randomized to one of two maintenance treatments (Zaharakis et al., 2008).

In initial analyses of outcomes from this study, there was a significant interaction effect ($p < .05$) between treatment condition and definition of *nonresponse* on measures of drinking frequency and severity during follow-up. Among the nonresponders randomized to the first criteria (i.e., 2 heavy drinking days), those who received both CBI and naltrexone had better drinking outcomes than those who received CBI and placebo. Conversely, in the nonresponders randomized to the more liberal definition (i.e., 5 heavy drinking days), those getting CBI plus placebo did better than those getting CBI plus naltrexone (Lynch et al., 2009). These results suggest that continuing to provide naltrexone to patients who have been stepped up to a more intensive behavioral intervention due to a poor initial response is more likely to be effective if the stepped care is provided relatively quickly after any drinking occurs. More reports from this intriguing study will be forthcoming over the next few years.

EXTENDED ADAPTIVE DISEASE MANAGEMENT FOR ALCOHOLISM

The second study discussed in this chapter is evaluating the effectiveness of an 18-month adaptive disease management protocol for alcohol-dependent patients who have achieved an initial positive response to intensive outpatient treatment (IOP), as evidenced by good attendance for 3 weeks. The adaptive protocol is built around telephone contacts that consist of an assessment of risk for relapse and brief problem-focused counseling. The calls, which are initiated while patients are still in IOP, are scheduled at 1-week intervals early in the protocol, with the frequency decreasing over time to one call per month. When risk levels increase, participants receive care that can include more frequent telephone sessions, several in-person sessions of MI (Miller & Rolnick, 2002), a course of relapse prevention (RP) at the clinic, or linkage back to the IOP. The primary control condition is IOP treatment as usual (TAU). A second control condition provides progress assessment and feedback on the same call schedule as the adaptive protocol but does not include counseling.

In the telephone-based adaptive treatment condition, the intensity of treatment remains low while patients are doing relatively well but is increased during periods of higher risk for relapse. Therefore, the intervention combines elements of low-intensity monitoring (Dennis, Scott, & Funk, 2003; Stout, Rubin, Zwick, Zywiak, & Bellino, 1999) and adaptive (L. M. Collins, Murphy, & Bierman, 2004; Lavori et al., 2000; Murphy et al., 2007) approaches. The protocol is designed to increase rates of sustained engagement and reduce costs relative to traditional, clinic-based treatment.

This intervention addresses most of the primary goals of the Chronic Care Model, as described by Wagner et al. (2001). This disease management model specifies regular, extended contact between patients and service providers; interventions to increase patient confidence and skills to manage chronic conditions (e.g., goal setting, identification of barriers to reaching goals, development of plans to overcome barriers); links to patient-oriented community resources; the use of accurate and timely patient data to monitor progress and guide interventions; and provision of support to facilitate improved self-management. Other investigators have also stressed the beneficial effects of regularly recording symptom severity and behaviors on health outcomes (Bandura, 1991; Febbraro & Clum, 1998), possibly because it serves as a prompt to maintain behavior change efforts. The Institute of Medicine's (2001) report on *Crossing the Quality Chasm* has also called for the use of methods of interaction between patient and caregiver other than face-to-face visits—such as the telephone—to facilitate ongoing contact in disease management programs.

Telephone Monitoring and Adaptive Counseling

Patients in this condition receive TAU plus a telephone-based intervention that commences after the 3rd week of IOP treatment. This intervention is an extension of a shorter (i.e., 12-week) telephone monitoring and counseling protocol that we used in a prior continuing care study

(McKay et al., 2004; McKay, Lynch, Shepard, & Pettinati, 2005; see also chap. 3, this volume).

General Protocol

Patients have one face-to-face session (60 minutes) early in their 4th week of IOP with the counselor who will be providing the telephone intervention. The purpose of this session is for the counselor to develop an initial rapport with the patient, explain the protocol, establish initial goals for the treatment, and provide a copy of the protocol workbook to the patient. Between therapeutic contacts, patients use the workbook to self-monitor risk and protective factors (e.g., any substance use, attendance at self-help) and progress toward the goals and objectives identified for that week.

The telephone portion of the protocol commences later in the same week. Telephone calls occur weekly for the first 8 weeks, twice monthly for the next 10 months, and once monthly for the final 6 months (for a total of 18 months). The patient and counselor decide who will initiate the calls; this decision is made on the basis of which approach is likely to yield the highest contact rate and is subject to review and change at later points. A toll-free number is available to the patients to help them complete calls when they do not have easy access to their own telephones. In both our prior telephone continuing care study (McKay, Lynch, et al., 2004) and this current alcohol disease management study, most patients have been able to access telephones consistently to make their calls, although sometimes this has meant calling in from recovery houses or the residences of friends or family members.

At the beginning of the call, the patient answers 10 brief questions about relapse risk and protective factors from the prior week (this assessment is described in the appendix). These data are combined to form a three-category risk score (i.e., low, moderate, or high), and information from this assessment is provided to the patients. For patients at low risk, patient and counselor go over the one or two goals that the patient is working on and the specific objectives that need to be accomplished to reach each goal. Any problems that were identified in the progress assessment are also addressed. In addition, reinforcement of positive behaviors and further encouragement for involvement in prorecovery activities are provided. For patients at moderate or high risk, some form of stepped care is recommended. Repeated failure on the part of the patient either to initiate the call or be reachable at the agreed-on call time becomes a focus of the intervention because it is likely to be indicative of wider problems with motivation and commitment to recovery. Patients are told that they should contact their telephone counselor between regularly scheduled sessions if they feel that they are suddenly at heightened risk for relapse or if they have actually used drugs or alcohol. A complete record of number of extra telephone contacts, length of each contact, and reason for the contact is obtained.

Although the telephone continuing care intervention is more convenient and less burdensome than many other continuing care interventions, not all patients to whom it is offered end up participating in it, as will be clear from data provided later in this chapter. Therefore, it is certainly not a panacea for attendance problems. Our studies feature intent-to-treat analyses, so the patients who are randomly assigned to a continuing care protocol are considered in the analyses, whether or not they receive any continuing care.

Adaptive Stepped-Care Component

The general principle underlying stepped care is a goal of maintaining the patient in the least intensive, least burdensome level of care whenever possible, reserving more intensive care for periods when the patient cannot be maintained at the lower level (M. B. Sobell & Sobell, 2000). If a patient's responses to the progress assessment indicate that he or she is at the moderate- or high-risk level, the stepped-care component of the adaptive protocol is triggered. If risk has risen to the moderate level and stayed there for several weeks, the frequency of telephone contacts is usually doubled for a period of 2 weeks. If risk returns to the low level after 2 weeks, the normal schedule of calls is resumed. If not, the increased call schedule is continued with reevaluation every 2 weeks.

If risk rises to the high level, the patient is asked to come into the research or clinical offices for a face-to-face MI session (Miller & Rollnick, 2002). The MI-based component is designed to allow for a broader reassessment than is possible with brief telephone contact and to address motivational concerns. The evaluation is organized around the dimensions of importance (i.e., motivation) and confidence (i.e., self-efficacy) for abstinence (Miller & Rollnick, 2002). The session begins with assessment of these two dimensions and depending on the patient's responses, the counselor proceeds in MI style either to increase the patient's perception of the importance of abstinence or to develop a workable plan to which the patient is willing to commit.

If the counselor and patient agree that a higher level of care is required, the patient may choose either to receive eight twice-weekly face-to-face CBT–RP sessions or to return to IOP. The CBT–RP sessions are based on a slightly modified version of the Carroll (1998) manual, which better places this intervention within the context of an adaptive, disease management protocol. In CBT–RP, patients learn to recognize the situations in which they are likely to use drugs (i.e., high-risk situations) and develop and practice new coping behaviors for those situations. Rehearsing new coping behaviors is thought to raise self-efficacy for handling them without using, which in turn is thought to reduce the likelihood of relapse (Marlatt & Gordon, 1985). The stepped-care protocol is described in more detail in the appendix.

Telephone Monitoring and Feedback

The telephone monitoring and feedback (TMF) condition was included to determine whether the positive effect of the extended telephone protocol over TAU—should such an effect be obtained—was due to the specific content of that intervention or simply to the provision of regular and extended contact with a counselor. Therefore, patients in this condition also have a face-to-face session with a telephone counselor in Week 4 and make telephone calls on the same schedule over the 18-month intervention period as those in the telephone monitoring and adaptive counseling (TMAC) condition. However, the telephone contacts consist only of the administration of the 10-item progress assessment instrument and brief feedback concerning results of the assessment:

1. *Low risk:* "You sound like you're doing very well. Let's talk again next week."
2. *Moderate risk:* "You're not drinking, but it looks like your motivation to remain abstinent has decreased and you are spending more time with people who are drinking. Perhaps it is time to consider going to more Alcoholics Anonymous meetings and making some other changes in your social life."
3. *High risk:* "You've begun to drink again and haven't been to an Alcoholics Anonymous meeting in several weeks. I strongly suggest that you contact your counselor and arrange to get back into treatment there or at some other program."

Study Methods and Assessments

Participants in the study complete follow-up assessments every 3 months over a 24-month follow-up. Data are gathered using structured and semistructured interviews (e.g., the Timeline Followback), self-administered questionnaires, collateral reports of substance use, blood measures of alcohol use, and urine toxicology tests for other drugs. All telephone and face-to-face therapeutic contacts in TMAC and TMF are audiorecorded and rated for adherence to the treatment manuals.

Preliminary Study Results

Two hundred and fifty-two participants were enrolled and randomized in this study. Approximately 24% of those randomized to TMAC or TMF never completed their initial face-to-face orientation session and therefore did not participate further in the extended telephone protocol. It should be noted that participants who did not complete their orientation session when it was originally scheduled were called repeatedly over the subsequent 6 months and sent letters in an effort to enroll them in the adaptive protocol. In some cases, participants did finally attend the orientation and began to complete telephone sessions. Call completion rates were high at first; for example, around 70% of all possible calls were completed in the 1st month. However, the completion rate for each possible call declined to approximately 40% by Month 3. Participants completed an average of about 11.5 calls in TMF and 8.9 calls in TMAC.

Predictors of Participation in Telephone Protocols

Preliminary analyses have been conducted to compare participants who attended their orientation session for the telephone protocols with those who did not. The variables that were entered into these analyses were treatment condition (i.e., TMAC vs. TMF), gender, education, and days of alcohol use, as well as Addiction Severity Index composite scores indicating problem severity at baseline (e.g., drug, employment, family and social, legal, medical, psychiatric). None of these variables was a significant predictor of attendance at the orientation session. It is possible that participants who did not attend their orientation were less motivated for additional treatment than the other study participants. Future analyses will examine a wider range of possible predictors.

Treatment Main Effects

Data from the 252 study participants were included in intent-to-treat outcome analyses, which examined alcohol use out to the 18-month follow-up (McKay, Lynch, Van Horn, et al., 2009). The results yielded a significant Treatment Group × Time interaction on one of the primary outcome measures—percentage days with any alcohol use in each quarter of the follow-up ($p = .01$). These results are presented in Figure 9.1. The results indicated effects favoring TMAC over TAU that increased in size over the 18-month follow-up. For example, in Months 13 through 15, percentage days of any alcohol use was 26% in TAU, 11% in TMF, and 3% in TMAC. Pair-wise comparisons indicated TMAC produced less frequent drinking than TAU at 9 and 12 months ($p < .05$), 15 months ($p < .001$), and 18 months ($p < .03$), and less frequent drinking than TMF at 6 months ($p = .01$). In addition, TMF produced less frequent drinking than TAU at 12 months ($p = .03$). Similar results were obtained with percentage days heavy drinking.

Outcomes on a second primary measure, total alcohol abstinence within each 3-month segment of the follow-up, are presented in Figure 9.2. With this dichotomous measure, there was a significant main effect for treatment condition ($p = .04$). Again at the 15-month follow-up, rates of any alcohol use in the prior 3 months were 52% in TAU, 41% in TMF, and 23% in TMAC. Difference of least squares means indicated lower rates of any drinking in TMAC relative to TAU across the follow-up ($p = .02$) and a trend in the comparison of TMF to TAU ($p = .08$).

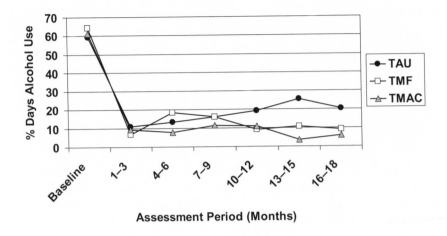

Figure 9.1. Frequency of alcohol use in each quarter of follow-up. Group × Time interaction: *p* = .01. TAU = treatment as usual; TMF = telephone monitoring and feedback; TMAC = telephone monitoring and adaptive counseling.

These results suggest that TEL is an effective method for sustaining good outcomes in alcohol-dependent patients receiving outpatient care. Shorter telephone calls that provide monitoring and feedback but no counseling appear to confer some benefit but are not as effective as longer calls that include counseling and stepped-care components.

Use of Stepped Care

Most of the stepped care that was successfully delivered was in the form of increased telephone contacts. It proved much more difficult to persuade participants who were struggling with increased craving, diminished confidence, or actual episodes of use to come back to the clinic for MI or CBT. Conversely, some participants stepped themselves up to higher intensities of treatment by going into inpatient facilities for detoxification, rehabilitation, or combined psychiatric and addiction treatment. A full report on utilization of stepped care is forthcoming.

EXTENDED ADAPTIVE DISEASE MANAGEMENT
FOR COCAINE DEPENDENCE

We are conducting a second extended continuing care study, this time focused on cocaine-dependent patients. The study is based on the adaptive disease management protocol that we tested in the alcohol study. However, there are a number of differences between the two studies with regard to treatment protocols. First, the new study includes two versions of TMAC

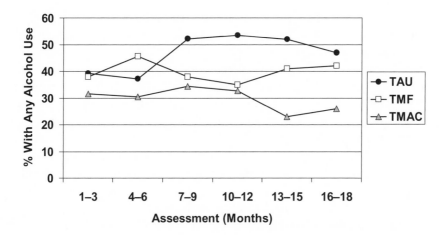

Figure 9.2. Alcohol use status in each quarter of follow-up. Main effect: TMAC < TAU, *p* = .02. TAU = treatment as usual; TMF = telephone monitoring and feedback; TMAC = telephone monitoring and adaptive counseling.

and drops the TMF condition. One version of TMAC is similar to that in the alcohol study, whereas the other includes incentives for sustained participation in the telephone calls ($10 gift certificate for each completed call, with a $10 bonus certificate for three consecutive calls) and for any recommended face-to-face stepped care (TMAC Plus). Incentives are also provided for cocaine-free urine samples, collected during face-to-face sessions with patients who have received recommended stepped care.

While participants are still attending IOP, the TMAC interventions also focus to a greater extent on supporting continued participation in IOP and on removing any barriers to participation, to avoid potential confusion on the part of the participant stemming from working with two counselors at once. We have modified the progress assessment done at the start of each call so that it seems less like "research" and yields information that better informs discussions focused on increasing retention and dealing with problems in the patients' lives. This new version of the progress assessment also provides more guidance to counselors on when and how to provide case management interventions, thereby guiding adaptive changes to the focus or content, rather than to the level of care or intensity, of treatment (i.e., *lateral* vs. *vertical* adaptation). These modifications are discussed in more detail in the appendix.

Several other modifications to the protocol were done to provide a better match for cocaine-dependent patients, who are more likely than alcohol-dependent patients to drop out early, engage in behaviors that increase risk of HIV, and remain at high risk for relapse over a prolonged period. Therefore, we are enrolling participants during their 2nd week in IOP, rather than waiting until the end of the 3rd week as we did in the alcohol study. An HIV risk reduction intervention and repeated HIV high-risk behavior assessments were also added to the TMAC orientation and call protocol. The face-to-face orientation has been expanded to two sessions to accommodate the HIV risk reduction intervention and to provide additional time for the telephone counselor and patient to establish initial connection and rapport. We are also placing a greater emphasis during the sessions on making sure that the issues of greatest concern and importance to the patient are always addressed on the calls. In that regard, patients are also allowed to come into the clinic for face-to-face sessions when they prefer to do so. Finally, the TMAC interventions have been extended to a full 24 months.

Preliminary results with the first 200 participants in the study, described in Figure 9.3, indicate that 81% of those randomized to the version of TMAC that includes incentives (i.e., TMAC Plus) completed the orientation sessions for that intervention versus 68% of those in the TMAC condition without incentives. Moreover, of those participants who completed their orientation sessions, 80% of all possible calls to date were successfully completed in TMAC Plus compared with 55% in TMAC (McKay, Long, Lynch, Van Horn, & Oslin, 2008). Initial analyses also suggest higher rates of participation in stepped care when it has been recommended by the counselors, compared with our alcohol telephone study described earlier in this chapter. Therefore, the new procedures that were instituted in this study appear to be substantially improving contact rates over what was achieved in the prior study. It is worth noting that although some of this improvement in contact rates is likely due to the use of incentives, we are still completing a high rate of calls in the condition that does not include incentives. The other modifications, which were designed to increase the strength of the counselor–patient connection at the start of the study and make the intervention itself of greater value to the patients, seem to have also increased motivation for extended participation in continuing care.

Interestingly, our initial examination of the session completion data has also indicated that the average length of the continuing care sessions in TMAC is greater than that in TMAC Plus by about 5 minutes (19.5 vs. 14.3 minutes). In addition, participants in TMAC were more likely to come into the office to complete their continuing care contact compared with those in TMAC Plus. These findings suggest that participants who are not receiving incentives for completing continuing care contacts are more engaged in the protocol, if they are participating at all, than those who are being incentivized.

CONCLUSION

We have learned several important lessons in these adaptive continuing care treatment studies. Despite the considerable "curb appeal" of adap-

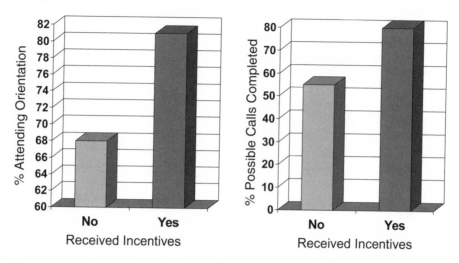

Figure 9.3. Impact of incentives on telephone continuing care participation.

tive interventions, engagement and sustained participation remain challenging issues. Not all patients want extended interventions, even if the burden is relatively low. Moreover, it can be difficult to get patients to accept stepped care, particularly when they are not doing well. Finally, telephone extended care models may be more likely to reach patients who are also doing other things to help support their recoveries, rather than patients who have stopped participating in self-help and other prorecovery activities.

Nonetheless, there is encouraging news here. Preliminary results from the extended alcohol continuing care study indicate superior treatment outcomes in the adaptive condition over the 18-month follow-up. The work of Scott and Dennis suggests that face-to-face contacts may facilitate higher rates of acceptance of stepped care (Dennis et al., 2003; Scott & Dennis, in press). Relatively low-level incentives also strongly increase rates of overall participation in telephone continuing care and appear to increase acceptance of stepped care recommendations. In addition, lateral modifications in which information obtained at the start of treatment sessions is used to adapt the content of that session while remaining in the same level of care may be more acceptable to patients than stepped care per se (i.e., recommendations to increase the intensity of treatment).

Finally, the preliminary results from the Oslin study provide information on two key methodological issues in adaptive treatment design (Lynch et al., 2009). First, it appears that the selection of a particular cutting point on a tailoring measure does matter in terms of the identification of responders and nonresponders, and the effectiveness of stepped care interventions. Second, it is possible to do sequential randomization in an addiction treatment study designed to develop an adaptive protocol and to retain most participants through the process. Chapter 10 provides detailed information for clinicians, program directors, and clinical researchers on how to design and implement adaptive treatment protocols for use in a clinic or practice. The material covers issues such as the identification of tailoring variables, selection of an appropriate menu of interventions, establishment of decision rules, and training of clinicians on the adaptive protocol.

10

DEVELOPING ADAPTIVE
TREATMENT PROTOCOLS
FOR CLINIC OR PRACTICE

Chapter 9 described in detail three adaptive treatment studies that are being conducted at the University of Pennsylvania and presented preliminary results from those studies. This chapter provides guidance to clinicians, program directors, and researchers who are interested in implementing adaptive treatments but who want to design and possibly evaluate their own algorithms. The material in this chapter outlines how to identify tailoring variables, select treatment options, and develop algorithms that link the two together to form an adaptive intervention. The role of patient choice or preference in the selection of treatment options, inclusion of medications, and training of clinicians is also covered.

As mentioned earlier in this book, many clinicians believe they make use of adaptive principles when delivering treatment to substance abusers. To some extent this is true; few therapists or counselors would persist in delivering exactly the same intervention to patients without paying any attention to how they are responding. Rather, most therapists will likely attempt to modify their approach to some degree if the patient is not responding to the current intervention. However, these modifications usually do not constitute a true adaptive intervention because they do not follow from a specified set of evidence-based tailoring variables, treatment options, and decision rules.

TAILORING VARIABLES

One of the key components of an adaptive protocol is the tailoring variable (or variables). Tailoring variables are selected to assess key markers of progress that are going to be used to construct the adaptive algorithm. There are several approaches to selecting tailoring variables; these are described in this section. However, it is important that tailoring variables have certain characteristics, no matter how they are selected. First, these variables must be clearly operationalized and as objective as possible. That is, they should be well-validated measures of specific constructs or behaviors. Second, if the tailoring variable is continuous or categorical with more than two response options, specific threshold or cutting scores need to be determined. Finally, the ideal tailoring variable will do more than simply predict outcome. Rather, it will predict better outcomes in one intervention compared with other interventions. A strong adaptive protocol specifies that when a specific value on a tailoring variable is observed, a patient who is doing poorly in Treatment A should be switched to Treatment B to improve outcome. For this to work, a tailoring variable is required that predicts little or no improvement in Treatment A but conversely predicts greater improvement in Treatment B. This is by far the hardest criterion to achieve in the selection of tailoring variables.

Recent findings concerning the clinical implications of having a positive cocaine urine toxicology test at intake to outpatient treatment illustrate this point. There is now good evidence that patients who have a positive urine screen at intake, indicating recent cocaine use, are at much higher risk of early dropout than those with a negative test (Alterman et al., 1997). This, of course, is not surprising; one would expect that patients who have managed to stop using cocaine for at least a few days before entering treatment would do better than those who were unable to do so. Does this mean that data from intake cocaine urine toxicology tests would make a good tailoring variable? Only if it can be shown that a particular treatment augmentation or switch would produce better outcomes for patients with positive urine tests than simply retaining them in standard care.

Hypothetical examples of tailoring variables and response in two treatment conditions are provided in the panels of Figure 10.1. In Panel A, higher scores on the tailoring variable predict poor outcome in both treatments, which indicates that outcomes of patients doing poorly in Treatment A will not improve if they are switched to Treatment B. This variable, although a good overall predictor, will not produce an effective adaptive algorithm. In

(A)

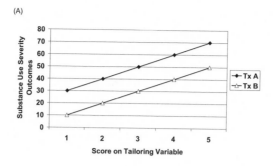

(B)

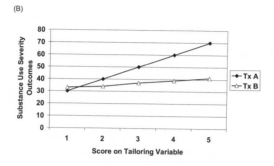

(C)

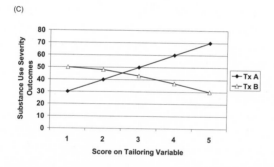

Figure 10.1. (A) Tailoring variable predicts outcome but not differential treatment response. (B) Tailoring variable predicts outcome and differential treatment response at high values. (C) Tailoring variable predicts outcome and differential treatment response at all values. Tx = treatment.

Panel B, higher scores on the tailoring variable predict worse outcome in Treatment A but not Treatment B, which suggests that outcomes might be improved if patients in Treatment A are switched to Treatment B if their scores on the tailoring variable increase at some point. Finally, in Panel C, lower scores on the tailoring variable predict better outcome in Treatment A, whereas higher scores predict better outcomes in Treatment B. This kind of complete cross-over effect makes for the strongest type of tailoring variable and is similar to the effect we observed in our telephone continuing care study (see chap. 8, Figure 8.4).

Theoretical Approach

With regard to methods for selecting tailoring variables, these markers might reflect the purported mechanisms of action of the treatment that is being delivered. For example, two important progress measures for 12-step-oriented treatment might be commitment to abstinence and attendance at 12-step meetings. These measures reflect the theoretical underpinnings of the 12-step approach and capture two of the important processes that are supposed to be happening during treatment—namely, that patients will become committed to total abstinence and will participate frequently in self-help meetings and related activities. Similarly, a therapist delivering a cognitive–behavioral therapy (CBT) or coping skills treatment might decide to monitor changes in coping behaviors and self-efficacy. In each of these two examples, failure to achieve the desired changes on the tailoring variables probably signals that the treatment is not working as intended and might trigger changes to the protocol, according to the rules of the adaptive algorithm.

Although working from a theory to select tailoring variables can have a number of important advantages over an atheoretical approach, there is one major caveat when it comes to behavioral interventions in the addictions. At this point, there is relatively little evidence that the purported "active ingredients," sometimes also referred to as *specific factors*, of various treatment approaches actually mediate treatment effects. For example, CBT is supposed to work by improving coping skills and motivational interviewing (MI) is intended to work by increasing readiness for change. However, there is at best only mixed evidence to support either of these supposed processes (Litt, Kadden, Cooney, & Kabela, 2003; Morgenstern & Longabaugh, 2000; Morgenstern & McKay, 2007). There is one exception to this general trend; it does appear that treatments designed to increase involvement in self-help programs do in fact accomplish this goal and that it is this increased involvement with self-help that mediates the effect of the treatment on subsequent outcomes (Longabaugh & Wirtz, 2001). Despite the lack of more convincing evidence for the specificity of mediation effects in addiction treatment, those interested in using the theoretical approach for selecting tailoring variables can certainly still base their selection on theory.

Outcome Measure Approach

Another approach to selecting tailoring variables involves directly monitoring the outcome of greatest interest during treatment. In addiction treatment, this is usually alcohol or drug use (or both). Under this approach, the therapist regularly assesses substance use during treatment and uses that information to decide whether treatment should be continued as currently delivered or modified in some way. Using the outcome measure as a tailoring variable has a number of advantages. Most important, it gets around the issue of whether the tailoring variable is a good marker of progress and is in fact related to outcome. There is ample evidence that substance use during treatment is a good predictor of substance use after treatment (Carroll et al., 1994; Higgins et al., 2000; McKay et al., 1999).

There are, however, two possible limitations inherent in focusing on substance use as a tailoring variable. First, because of social desirability issues, asking directly about use may invite inaccurate reporting. Second, ignoring process measures and focusing directly on substance use precludes gathering information about what might be going wrong with the treatment. For example, in a CBT treatment, focusing strictly on substance use will not indicate where treatment is breaking down in a patient who is exhibiting poor progress—whether the problem is low motivation, inability to recognize high-risk situations, failure to learn new coping skills, or the emergence of unforeseen relapse triggers.

McLellan et al. (2005) also recommended that other domains be considered for monitoring during addiction treatment. These investigators highlighted what they refer to as the other three traditional outcome domains in addiction treatment: personal health, social function, and public health and safety. Personal health refers to medical and psychiatric problem severity, social function to the quality of interpersonal relations and employment, and public safety to criminal behavior and HIV high-risk behavior. The idea here is that by monitoring patients' status in these additional areas, clinicians would be in a better position to arrange for adjunctive treatment services when appropriate to augment basic addiction-focused treatment. McLellan et al. referred to this procedure as continuous recovery monitoring (CRM). The feasibility of frequent monitoring of progress in treatment through interactive voice response (IVR) has also been explored by T. L. Simpson, Kivlahan, Bush, and McFall (2005).

Empirical Approach

A third approach to selecting tailoring variables is to make use of existing data, either from published studies or a clinic database. For example, data that could be used to identify treatment process measures that predict outcome might be a good potential source of tailoring variables. This approach is not necessarily atheoretical, in that the theories on which treatments are based can be a valuable guide on where to look for possible tailoring variables. However, it places a greater emphasis on the use of empirical processes to select such variables. One of the advantages of the empirical approach is that it allows for the possibility of combining several relatively weak tailoring variables into one potentially more effective composite or index.

The first University of Pennsylvania telephone-based continuing care (TEL) study, described in chapter 8 of this volume, provides one example of the empirical approach to selecting tailoring variables. In this study, we were interested in identifying variables that would predict which graduates of a 4-week intensive outpatient program (IOP) would do best in each of three possible step-down continuing care treatments: group counseling, individualized relapse prevention, and telephone-based counseling. Our initial working hypothesis was that patients with greater problem severity at the start of IOP and those who made poorer progress toward achieving the goals of the program would require more intensive continuing care, whereas those with lower problem severity and those who made better progress toward program goals would do equally well, if not better, in lower intensity continuing care.

With regard to pre-IOP problem severity, we focused on two factors: current dependence on both alcohol and cocaine and a diagnosis of lifetime major depression. These variables were selected because of a large research literature in which the co-occurrence of alcohol and cocaine dependence and psychiatric problems has consistently predicted worse outcomes. We thought that patients with these characteristics would likely do better in the two more intensive face-to-face treatments, compared with the less intensive telephone continuing care intervention. We did not consider other pre-IOP variables, primarily because we assumed that they would be less useful than more proximal measures assessed during IOP.

The measures that assessed progress during IOP were selected after discussions with IOP program directors and counselors and a review of published literature on traditional, 12-step-oriented treatment programs. Not surprisingly, the first goals that were nominated were the achievement of initial abstinence from alcohol and drugs during IOP. Other goals that were frequently mentioned were regular attendance at self-help meetings, commitment to abstinence, ability to cope with high-risk situations, readiness to change, social support for recovery, and reduced psychiatric symptom severity. We were able to operationalize all these constructs with measures from the study, with two exceptions. Our measure of social support was a general measure of perceived support from friends and family, rather than a measure of support specifically for abstinence or recovery. Also, a measure of perceived ability to cope with high-risk situations (i.e., self-efficacy) was available but not a direct measure of coping abilities. These constructs were measured at the end of the 4-week IOP program.

In the first analyses, each potential tailoring variable was examined separately (McKay, Lynch, Shepard, Morgenstern, et al., 2005). The analyses evaluated the overall predictive power of each measure, but the real test was whether the measures interacted with treatment condition to predict outcome. Because the primary focus of the analyses was to identify factors that were associated with good or poor outcome in the telephone condition, relative to the two face-to-face treatments, the possible moderator effects of each potential tailoring variable were tested through two focused contrasts that were carved out of the overall Treatment Condition × Tailoring Variable interaction term: group counseling versus TEL and relapse prevention (RP) versus TEL. All in all, 40 potential moderator effects were tested (10 Tailoring Variables × 2 Contrasts × 2 Outcome Measures).

Given the number of tests that were performed, one would have expected a couple of findings to reach the .05 level of significance by chance alone. However, of the 40 analyses that were performed, only one interaction effect was significant at the .05 level. In patients with any alcohol use during IOP, group counseling produced higher percentage days abstinent than TEL as well as a trend toward higher rates of total abstinence. Notably, only 4 of the other 38 interactions yielded a p value less than .20. This suggested that there was little evidence that these measures were going to be effective tailoring variables in an algorithm designed to steer IOP graduates into the most appropriate form of continuing care. The other limitation in the results with the individual measures was that the one significant finding provided no information on which patients would be most appropriate for the low-intensity telephone condition. This is because the plot of the interaction effect showed that all three treatments produced equivalent outcomes with patients who did not drink during IOP, whereas group counseling continuing care was more effective than TEL for those who drank at all.

Developing Composite Tailoring Variables

Despite these disappointing findings, it was possible that positive (i.e., poor prognosis) scores on a number of these indicators might together predict poorer outcomes in TEL, relative to RP or group counseling. We therefore developed a composite measure of the risk indicators that consisted of a simple sum of dichotomized versions of seven of the tailoring measures. The seven items that formed the composite risk indicator measure were (a) any alcohol use in the prior 30 days, (b) any cocaine use in the prior 30 days, (c) current dependence at entrance to IOP on both alcohol and cocaine, (d) attendance at fewer than 12 self-help meetings during the prior 30 days, (e) score on the social support measures that was below the median in the study sample, (f) abstinence goal less stringent than total abstinence, and (g) self-efficacy score of less than 80%. Each item was scored either 1 (indicating higher risk) or 0 (McKay, Lynch, Shepard, Morgenstern, et al., 2005).

Lifetime major depression and Addiction Severity Index psychiatric composite were not included in the composite risk indicator because they were essentially unrelated to substance use outcomes and showed no evidence of matching effects. With regard to motivation, commitment to abstinence was included, rather than readiness to change, because it was more closely linked to IOP goals and would be much easier for clinicians to score and use given that it consists of only one item. The cutting score for self-help attendance was based on standard practices in typical IOPs, whereas the cutting score for self-efficacy was determined by a review of research findings on posttreatment self-efficacy scores in addiction treatment studies. A median split was used with the sum of the social support measures because of a lack of clinical or research data on which to base the cutting score. Rates of endorsement of each item ranged from a low of 13% for any alcohol use in the prior 30 days to a high of 51% for an abstinence goal less stringent than total abstinence. Patients averaged a total score of 2.50 (standard deviation [SD] = 1.36), and scores on the measure were well distributed (see chap. 8, Figure 8.3). Variables were coded so that higher scores on the composite risk indicator signified poorer progress in treatment.

Regression analyses were done with the composite risk indicator measure to ascertain the main effect for this measure and whether it was a predictor of differential response to the three continuing care treatments. The dependent measure in the analyses was total abstinence (yes–no) within each 3-month segment of the follow-up. In the regression, the IOP composite risk indicator measure was highly significant ($p < .0001$), with higher scores associated with lower abstinence rates. In the two focused contrasts carved out of the Treatment Condition × Performance Score interaction, the group counseling versus TEL contrast was significant (estimate = .38, odds ratio [OR] = 1.47, $p = .045$), whereas the RP versus TEL contrast was not (estimate = .22, OR = 1.25, $p = .25$). Data presented in Figure 8.4 (see chap. 8) indicate that as scores on the composite risk indicator measure increased, the probability of abstinence during each quarter declined. However, this effect was more pronounced in the TEL condition than in the group counseling condition, which accounted for the significant contrast effect. Generally, patients with scores of 3 or less on the measure did better in TEL than in group counseling, whereas those with scores above 3 did better in group counseling than in TEL (McKay, Lynch, Shepard, Morgenstern, et al., 2005; McKay, Lynch, Shepard, & Pettinati, 2005). The same general pattern was found in the comparisons between TEL and RP, although the difference between slopes was not as pronounced.

Our experience with selecting and testing possible tailoring variables illustrates the importance of subjecting potential measures to empirical tests, to determine whether they in fact perform as expected. Reliance on expert opinion and prior research findings can be extremely useful in narrowing the field of possible measures down to a reasonable number, but an empirical test is necessary to confirm the utility of the measures. Ideally, what one is looking for is a measure that predicts a true crossover type of interaction in which high scores on the measure predict better outcomes in Treatment A than Treatment B, and low scores predict the opposite (i.e., better outcomes in Treatment B than Treatment A; see Panel C of Figure 10.1). However, a measure that at least predicted differential outcomes at one level or score, and equivalent outcomes at another level, can still be useful in setting up an adaptive protocol (see Panel B of Figure 10.1). For example, a clinic might discover that when patients' self-efficacy level drops below 50% confidence in being able to cope successfully without using a substance, it makes sense to augment their standard group treatment with individual coping skills treatment.

The results of our study also highlight the possibility that combining several tailoring measures might produce a stronger adaptive algorithm than relying on a single measure. An important question, of course, is, How should clinicians go about putting together such an index? How many variables should be included? Should they all count equally, or should some be weighted more heavily than others? With all the possible choices to be made, the process can seem daunting. In our case, we opted for a basic approach, which involved selecting the measures that looked at least somewhat promising in the univariate analyses, dichotomizing them, and simply adding up the scores without weighting any of the measures (i.e., each measure contributed equally to the scale). Subsequent efforts to refine our scale via more complicated statistical procedures have not produced a revised scale with greater power to determine which patients do best in TEL and group counseling continuing care (S. Murphy, personal communication, July 2006).

Establishing Cutting Scores With Continuous Tailoring Variables

Regardless of the approach taken to selecting and testing potential tailoring variables, at some point cutting scores must be selected in order for the measures to be used in adaptive protocols. In cases in which the measure in question is already categorical rather than continuous, this poses no problems. However, in the case of continuous measures, how does one make a choice? For example, a clinician might devise a stepped care protocol that begins with two MI sessions and bibliotherapy, followed by weekly monitoring of alcohol use. The protocol calls for augmenting this intervention with CBT if it does not appear to be working with a particular patient. The clinician selects number of days of heavy drinking over the 1st month as his tailoring variable. The question is, How many heavy drinking days must occur before augmentation with CBT is recommended to the patient? Specifically, should CBT be added relatively quickly, perhaps after 1 or 2 days of heavy drinking, or should the patient be given a few weeks in initial protocol before CBT is added, even if heavy drinking continues?

When faced with a question such as this, a clinician or program may decide that clinical experience and common sense, coupled with existing reports in the literature, are sufficient for deciding on a cutting score for the tailoring measure. In this example, for instance, the clinician may decide that the possible negative consequences associated with continued heavy drinking outweigh any possible disadvantages of stepped care. In that case, a more conservative cutting score would be adopted (e.g., add CBT if patient has more than 1 heavy drinking day within 4 weeks). However, clinical experience and common sense may not steer the clinician or program in one direction or the other, and there may be no findings in the literature that bear on the particular question at hand. In these circumstances, it may be advisable to consider the possibility of conducting a small study to determine the optimal cutting point.

The ideal study of this type would involve randomizing patients to two or more possible cutting scores and examining whether this makes any difference with regard to outcomes. It is important to remember that outcomes in this case are not some distal measure of drinking behavior (e.g., percentage days abstinent at 12 months). Rather, the outcomes should be proximal measures of engagement in treatment and substance use that are gathered during treatment. Regarding the example here, appropriate outcomes to consider might include percentage of patients stepped up to CBT who actually attended CBT, number of CBT sessions attended, and number of heavy drinking days over the first 2 months in treatment. If the cutting score makes a difference, we would observe higher rates of acceptance of stepped care, more days in stepped care, and fewer heavy drinking days with patients for whom changes in treatment were driven by one cutting score compared with the other.

Although randomization is ideal for demonstrating causality, it is not always possible to randomize within a particular practice or clinic. Therefore, a practitioner or clinic might consider a quasi-experimental study instead. For example, 20 consecutive patients might be treated using one cutting score and the next 20 with the other cutting score. Again, the important question is whether different cutting scores on a tailoring variable make a difference in short-term patient outcomes. If such a difference emerges when quasi-experimental methods are used, it would still make sense to proceed with the cutting score that produced the best outcomes, rather than waiting for results from a study with a stronger design.

MENU OF CLINICAL INTERVENTIONS

The second component of an adaptive treatment algorithm is a menu of clinical interventions or services. The key requirement here is that the clinical services in the menu are meaningfully different on at least one dimension, such as frequency, intensity, modality, content, theoretical orientation, and so forth. For an adaptive strategy to work, the treatment options must be different enough that failure in one treatment approach will not strongly predict failure in all the other possible approaches in the menu. For example, an algorithm that steps up patients who are not doing well in a one session per week outpatient program to two sessions per week of the same treatment is unlikely to be effective, nor are algorithms that switch patients between two variants of CBT. For that matter, there are real questions whether switching nonresponders over to another individually focused talk therapy if they are not responding to the first treatment provided will result in a higher rate of response. Rather, it may be necessary to switch to or augment care with a very different approach.

Possible Augmentations for Nonresponders

What might such a change in treatment look like? Here are several possible examples of treatment augmentations, all for patients who have not experienced a good response to standard group-based, outpatient addiction treatment:

- add motivational interviewing in individual sessions,
- add adjunctive service designed to address co-occurring problem (e.g., marital therapy, psychiatric care),
- add active case management in individual sessions,
- add a medication to combat craving or decrease the rewarding effects of alcohol or drugs,
- add incentives for abstinence through a contingency management protocol, or
- increase level of care (e.g., outpatient to residential).

Possible Treatment Switches for Nonresponders

Unfortunately, many patients who are not doing well in a particular level or type of care are not often interested in "more treatment." This can be due to a number of reasons, including flagging motivation for treatment, dislike of the standard addiction specialty care approach that is heavily based on 12-step principles and is abstinence-oriented, competing family and employment responsibilities, and so forth. Therefore, it may also be worth considering changes to standard group-based treatment that involve switching to either different or even less intensive interventions or otherwise switching the content of the intervention. Such modifications might include,

- switch to a watchful waiting or self-change approach in which patient attempts to reduce substance use while being monitored regularly by the counselor;
- switch to an individualized, low-intensity approach such as MI, followed by regular monitoring;
- switch to a medical approach that combines primary care–based monitoring with a medication such as naltrexone; or
- switch to some other type of treatment that is more compatible with the patient's beliefs or preferences.

Of course, it is easier for a full-service clinic to provide a range of possible treatment modifications than it is for a solo practitioner to do so. However, even clinics with more extensive resources may have trouble getting reimbursed for some treatment switches or augmentations, particularly to more medication-oriented interventions or to less intensive behavioral treatments. For example, in many locations, intensive outpatient treatment is reimbursed at a much higher rate than standard outpatient treatment, and there are limitations on how many individual counseling sessions can be provided in lieu of group counseling. Moreover, not all effective medications are covered by health insurance policies. These funding structures make it difficult to deviate from the IOP or standard outpatient approach.

Given these limitations, it is probably advisable for clinics and practitioners attempting to implement adaptive treatment protocols to work toward identifying one or two meaningfully different treatment options that could actually be provided to patients who do not respond to standard care. Because patients exhibiting a poor response to standard care are at high risk of dropout, switching them to a lower intensity intervention that they will continue to participate in may not result in a loss of revenue.

Adaptive algorithms can also be used to specify the content of interventions. In switching from one type of intervention to another—say from a 12-step-based treatment to CBT or from individual to couples-based treatment—one clearly changes the content of the intervention, even if the frequency and duration of the sessions stay the same. However, adaptive algorithms could also be developed that specify less dramatic shifts with a particular therapeutic approach. These might include when to focus on biased beliefs versus coping deficits in CBT or on empathy versus more directive techniques in MI. For such changes in content to truly constitute an adaptive intervention, they would need to be linked to specific values on a tailoring variable, perhaps assessed at the start of each treatment session. Of course, research would be required to determine whether an adaptive algorithm that drove changes in session content actually produced improvements in outcome.

Individual Versus Group Treatment and Adaptive Protocols

Several comments are in order concerning group versus individual treatment. Because adaptive treatment is individualized on the basis of progress over time, one might assume that it has to be delivered within the context of individual therapy or counseling. This is actually not the case. A number of the adaptive interventions described in this book have been done with patients in group counseling interventions. It may be desirable to include individual therapy, such as case management, as a step-up treatment for patients who are not doing well in standard group therapy or counseling, but even this is certainly not required. The key point is that adaptive protocols need to include a menu of intervention options, so that treatment can be modified on the basis of progress or the lack thereof.

Adaptive Treatment for Responders

What about patients who do well in treatment? Is it worth considering adaptive protocols for them as well? What kinds of step-down treatments have proved effective? Before these questions are considered, it is first worth considering another issue—whether a patient who is doing well should simply stay in the same intervention for a prolonged period of time. There is now evidence, for example, that depressed patients who respond well to a particular treatment are best served by staying on that treatment for an extended period (Jarrett et al., 2001). Might the same be true of a person with alcohol dependence who is doing well in IOP—why not keep the patient in IOP? The main issue here is whether there are diminishing returns associated with keeping a patient at a higher level of care for longer periods of time. For example, longer stays in intensive treatment increase the cost of treatment—to whoever funds it, of course, but also to the patient if it interferes with other important life roles such as employment or parenting. There is also some possibility that patients' frustration with the demands of extended high-intensity treatment might lead to diminished participation in subsequent continuing care, although there is no research evidence to indicate whether that is true.

Unfortunately, there is little evidence concerning how long the initial treatment should be provided to give the patient a good shot at a sustained recovery or how long patients should be kept at various levels of care before a step-down can be considered. Correlational data suggest that patients who stay in treatment for at least 90 days seem to do better, but these data do not differentiate primary versus step-down care. Moreover, they are likely biased to some degree by self-selection processes. The optimal length of treatment may also vary as a function of the nature of the addiction and other characteristics of the patient and his or her social environment. Many clinicians who work with patients with long histories of opiate addiction, for example, believe that these patients should stay on methadone for extended periods of time, long after they have become stabilized on the medication. In that regard, one of the studies reviewed earlier indicated that sustained provision of methadone led to better outcomes than shorter durations followed by gradual detoxification (Sees et al., 2000).

Our telephone continuing care study, described in detail in prior chapters, is perhaps the only study at this point that provides empirically based guidelines for how progress in one level of care (e.g., IOP) can be used to select the most appropriate step-down treatment. However, that study had several limitations that raise questions about generalizability. First, the IOPs that were included in the study were 4 weeks in duration, and patients graduated to step-down care as long as they were still attending and were abstinent in the 4th week (those who were using in that week were given an additional week or 2 to achieve abstinence before step down). Because of this, our algorithm development could focus only on the question of what treatment would be best to deliver next and could not address the question of when to alter treatment. Many publicly funded IOPs now have longer potential maximum lengths of stay, leading to the need to address both the "what" and "when" issues when putting together an algorithm. Second, our study essentially ignored those who dropped out of IOP before graduation. One might argue that it is these patients who are in most need of an adaptive continuum of care, because they have failed to get engaged in treatment.

The American Society of Addiction Medicine placement and continuation criteria, described in chapter 6, provide some guidance on when patients have achieved sufficient reductions in problem severity to warrant stepping down to lower levels of care. These continuation criteria suggest that patients be maintained at the current level of care, until problem severity levels on all six ASAM dimensions have dropped below specified criteria. However, these decision rules have not been validated in any controlled studies. Clearly, there are many unanswered questions at this point concerning when patients can be stepped down to lower intensity interventions within an adaptive algorithm and what types of interventions are likely to be effective. More research is needed to address the following issues:

1. When are residential patients ready to step down to outpatient treatment?
2. When are IOP patients ready to step down to standard outpatient treatment?
3. When are outpatients who are also attending self-help ready to continue on self-help alone?
4. When are patients receiving both behavioral and pharmacological interventions ready to step down to only one intervention?
5. What kinds of step-down care produce the highest rates of sustained participation and lowest rates of substance use?

DECISION RULES

The decision rules in an adaptive protocol link the tailoring variables and the menu of clinical intervention options into one algorithm. The finished algorithm will read like a series of "if–then" statements:

> If a score of greater than X on the tailoring variable Y is obtained, then augment Treatment A with Treatment B. If a score of less than X on the tailoring variable Y is obtained, continue to provide Treatment A for another 4 weeks and re-assess.

If we think of two possible broad outcomes on the tailoring variables—one indicating nonresponse and the other indicating positive response—there is a fairly limited set of possible types of adaptation:

- Nonresponders
  - Step up (e.g., outpatient to IOP or residential)
  - Modality change (e.g., CBT to medication)
  - Lateral move (e.g., CBT to TSF)
  - Change in content within a particular intervention
  - Step down (e.g., IOP to telephone monitoring)
- Responders
  - Reduce frequency of intervention (e.g., IOP to outpatient)
  - Change to lower burden intervention (e.g., outpatient to periodic checkups or e-treatment)

Again, the decision rules that link specific scores on tailoring variables to modifications in treatment are arrived at through one of two processes, either expert consensus or an experimental study. Regardless of how the algorithm is developed, it is advisable to conduct studies to evaluate how well it is working. These studies need not involve randomization, as long as good baseline data are available on the outcome measure. For example, data from the information management system of a treatment program might document that the 60-day retention rate in the program's IOP has consistently been approximately 50% for the past 2 years. After the program has introduced a new adaptive algorithm designed to reengage patients who drop out early, the 60-day retention rate can be reexamined to see whether it has gone up a clinically significant amount. If the adaptive algorithm has not accomplished its goal, it can be modified with the hope of improving performance and evaluated again with the next group of patients. This procedure has been referred to as *continuous quality improvement*.

ROLE OF PATIENT PREFERENCE

There is increasing recognition of the importance of patient preferences and choices when it comes to treatment engagement, retention, and outcomes (Institute of Medicine, 2006; Krahn & Naglie, 2008; Wagner et al., 2001). Some patients are committed to 12-step-focused, abstinence-oriented programs, whereas others want nothing to do with that kind of treatment. Some patients prefer medication over intensive behavioral interventions, whereas others have no confidence in pills and instead prefer talk therapy. When patients come to a traditional specialty care addiction program, there is at least some chance that they are open to that type of treatment. However, individuals whose substance use disorder has been identified while they are receiving care for something else (e.g., medical care, emergency department) may be considerably less open to traditional abstinence-oriented approaches. Providing treatment options to these people may be particularly important.

With regard to continuing care, patients may differ in what kinds of treatment they are willing to commit to following the completion of their initial phase of care. Some, for example, may have greater employment or family responsibilities and will prefer a more flexible approach that does not require weekly visits to the clinic. Patient preference can also be factored into adaptive algorithms, particularly to improve outcomes in nonresponders. For example, an adaptive algorithm might call for providing a patient with the choice of several possible treatments options, should he drop out of standard group-based continuing care relatively early. At this point, there is virtually no research on the impact of patient choice in addiction treatment. However, one can make a convincing case for the importance of considering what he or she is willing to try when attempting to deliver treatment to a patient who does not appear to want whatever treatment was offered first.

ADAPTIVE MEDICATION PROTOCOLS

With diseases such as cancer, depression, and hypertension, there are multiple medications for clinicians to choose from. Moreover, there are usually efficacious choices within several classes of drugs. Adaptive protocols in these areas are therefore able to specify switches or augmentations within a drug class or between classes for patients who do not respond to the first medication prescribed. This range of choices was evident in the Sequenced Treatment Alternatives to Relieve Depression (STAR*D) study for depression, described in chapter 7, in which the algorithms considered included switching or augmenting a first-line selective serotonin reuptake inhibitor (SSRI) with other SSRIs or with medications from other classes.

Unfortunately, as of this writing, there are relatively few options in efficacious medications for addiction. There are three Food and Drug Administration–approved medications for alcohol dependence: disulfiram (Antabuse), naltrexone (Revia), and acamprosate (Campral). Although these three medications appear to work through different mechanisms, there is no evidence thus far that any one works in patients who do not respond to one of the others, and one large study found no advantage to augmenting naltrexone with acamprosate (Anton et al., 2006). An injectable form of naltrexone, Vivitrol, may be useful for patients who respond well to oral naltrexone but do not stay on the medication or may be more effective initially than oral naltrexone with some patients; however, studies on this topic have not yet been performed.

Three medications are also available for opiate-dependent patients—methadone, buprenorphine, and naltrexone. As described in chapter 8, there is already evidence to support the effectiveness of an adaptive algorithm that starts patients on buprenorphine and moves them to methadone only if they are not doing well on the first medication (Kakko et al., 2007). The evidence for effective medications for cocaine or methamphetamine dependence is even weaker (O'Brien & McKay, 2006). There are no algorithms currently available that specify adaptive medication protocols for stimulant disorders.

TRAINING CLINICIANS TO USE THE ADAPTIVE ALGORITHM

Training clinicians in the use of an adaptive algorithm should start with a review of the algorithm, how it was derived, and what it is supposed to accomplish. A manual that clearly spells out the tailoring variables, treatment options, and decision rules in the adaptive algorithm is a must. Recordings or transcripts of sessions that illustrate correct and incorrect applications of the algorithm can be extremely helpful in training clinicians to use it properly.

In our experience, training seasoned clinicians to follow an adaptive algorithm consistently can be difficult, even when it possesses considerable face validity. Many of the problems seem to center on the clinician's perception that although the algorithm is generally good, decisions regarding the treatment of a particular patient should be made differently. Most experienced clinicians trust their clinical judgment more than a score on a tailoring variable. For example, a clinician may want to step up a patient to a higher level of care, even though the patient's score on the tailoring variable does not indicate that this should be done at that time (e.g., "I know Joe's score does not indicate we should do anything now, but I'm picking up some other indicators not covered by that measure that make me worried he's about to relapse"). Or a clinician may agree with the tailoring variable that an adaptive change is in order but feel that a different type of change would be most effective (e.g., "Marcia has started drinking again and clearly needs a change in her treatment. I know the protocol calls for adding naltrexone at this point, but I really believe that she'll respond better if I double the frequency of her CBT sessions").

Also, clinicians may not want to send a marginally responsive patient to another form of treatment if it involves giving the case over to another provider (e.g., "I know that the protocol says we need to switch Joan from medication management to a more intensive program at the clinic because she's had another bout of heavy drinking, but I really think I can manage her drinking at this level of care if we give her a little more time to stabilize").

To determine how well clinicians are following adaptive protocols, it is necessary for the clinic to maintain accurate and complete data on tailoring variable scores over time, whether the algorithm-driven change in treatment was specified when the tailoring variable indicated it should be, and whether the clinician and patient followed through with the specified change. Careful attention to the collection and regular examination of such data will indicate how often clinicians are deviating from the "if–then" statements of the algorithm. These data should be discussed in supervision either to reinforce proper use of the algorithm decision rules or to address its incorrect use. Additional supervision will be most important for clinicians who are not getting good outcomes with the adaptive protocol.

It should be noted that in our adaptive treatment studies, we do allow clinicians some latitude in following the protocol as long as they thoroughly document their reasons for deviating from the explicit decision rules. Such information is actually quite useful in guiding future modifications to adaptive protocols to improve their effectiveness because it can flag where the algorithm breaks down.

CONCLUSION

Outside of the context of a research study, in which treatments must be delivered according to what are usually fairly fixed protocols, most clinicians attempt to be flexible in their approach with patients. If the treatment provided is not working as intended and the patient is not getting better, adjustments are made over time until a better response is obtained. The procedures described in this chapter can be used to help clinicians standardize and—it is hoped—improve the effectiveness of this process of adjusting treatment while it is being provided.

Perhaps the most important take-home message is that adaptive protocols that clinicians develop for their clinic or practice can be improved through repeated assessments of their efficacy on measures of short-term outcomes, such as attendance or substance use. If the protocol does not appear to be performing as expected, the clinician or program director can institute modifications and determine whether outcomes improve with the next cohort of patients. Of course, for this process to be effective, the modifications to the existing protocol need to be delivered consistently. Therefore, it is highly recommended that any modifications to the adaptive protocol be clearly described in a revised treatment manual and adherence to the modified protocol monitored carefully.

To engage in this process of developing, implementing, evaluating, and improving an adaptive intervention, clinicians or clinics need to be able to collect data on several variables. These include scores on the selected tailoring variable(s), clinician recommendations regarding treatment modifications in response to scores on the tailoring variable(s), the patient's response to the recommendation (e.g., whether patient attended recommended stepped care), and short-term outcomes (e.g., treatment attendance, substance use). These data should be reviewed on a regular basis to inform discussions of whether the adaptive protocol is working as intended. The input of all clinicians in a particular clinic or practice is important to the process of evaluating and modifying an adaptive protocol.

Chapter 11 addresses some of the challenges that clinicians and investigators will face in designing, implementing, and evaluating adaptive protocols. These include problems with compliance and retention, lack of truly different treatment alternatives, incorporation of patient preference, and analysis of study data.

11

CHALLENGES IN DESIGNING, IMPLEMENTING, AND EVALUATING ADAPTIVE PROTOCOLS

The rationale for adaptive treatment is compelling, and the studies reviewed here provide a reasonably convincing case for the effectiveness of this approach. However, a number of challenges still need to be addressed. Most of these are common to all approaches to addiction treatment, whereas some are more specific to adaptive models of care. The issues that are discussed in this chapter are problems with retention and compliance, lack of viable treatment alternatives, the tension between results at the levels of group and individual, and timing of the assessment of tailoring variables.

Attempts to evaluate adaptive disease management interventions can also raise several thorny issues that are not encountered in more traditional randomized controlled trials. For example, most controlled clinical trials strive to deliver the same intervention to all participants within a particular treatment condition, whereas adaptive treatments are designed to change over time in response to changes in the participants. Therefore, no two participants are likely to receive exactly the same intervention. In this chapter, new research designs and statistical approaches for examining treatment main effects and identifying key treatment process variables are described.

PROBLEMS WITH RETENTION AND COMPLIANCE

The idea of adaptive treatment is predicated on the assumption that patients will comply with recommended changes to their treatments. In some areas of medicine, this is a relatively safe assumption. For example, individuals with hypertension who are not responding adequately to an initial medication will usually accept an augmentation in the form of a second medication as long as side effects do not increase. In fact, one way to reduce the incidence of side effects when a first medication is not achieving the desired outcome is to add a low to moderate dose of a second medication, rather than increase the dose of the first medication. Similarly, on the basis of the results of the Sequenced Treatment Alternatives to Relieve Depression study (STAR*D; Rush et al., 2006), a patient with depression who does not achieve remission is likely to be willing to try augmenting that medication or switching to an entirely different medication.

However, we are often in entirely different territory with substance abuse patients who are not getting better early in treatment. Frequently, these patients have lost some or most of their commitment to treatment and recovery and may have started to use alcohol or drugs again. They may be difficult to keep engaged at all, let alone in stepped care, which includes augmentations or intensifications to standard treatment. For example, a patient who started treatment in an intensive outpatient program but has not managed to achieve initial abstinence may not be willing to participate in a more intensive program such as residential treatment, unless compelled to do so to avoid criminal justice consequences or loss of custody of children. Therefore, adaptive continuing care protocols in the addictions need to consider various ways to motivate struggling patients to accept modifications to treatment.

Make Treatment More Appealing

One approach to improve retention in adaptive algorithms involves finding ways to make the modification more appealing to the patient. For example, failure at one level of care need not automatically lead to recommendations for more treatment. A patient might not be ready for the time commitment and emphasis on total abstinence that comes along with traditional intensive outpatient program (IOP) treatment but would be willing to participate in a less intensive intervention that allowed for substance use goals other than total abstinence. The *alcohol care management* intervention described in chapter 12 is an example of such an intervention. Some treatment programs have begun to use *pretreatment groups* to manage patients who are not willing to make the commitment to more intensive, abstinence-oriented treatment. It may even be possible to follow such patients by telephone for a period of time in an effort to maintain some degree of therapeutic contact and capitalize on the emergence of "teachable mo-ments" in which the patient will be more open to suggestions to reenter standard treatment.

The prior example raises the issue of the potential role of patient preference or choice in the process of modifying treatment. There is usually little room for patients' preferences for treatment, either in real-world clinics or in research studies. In research, for example, participants are typically randomized to one of several treatment options without regard to—and sometimes in contradiction with—their actual preferences. The patient is expected to take the treatment he or she is assigned to, and failure to do so results in a protocol violation. Similarly, patients seeking treatment in the community often have little choice in what they receive; rather, treatment selection is made on the basis of placement criteria like that of the American Society of Addiction Medicine, treatment availability, or insurance coverage. However, choice with regard to type of intervention may be an extremely important factor in the willingness of patients to seek and subsequently accept further care when they have experienced relapses during treatment (Dwight-Johnson et al., 2001; Institute of Medicine, 2006; Krahn & Naglie, 2008; McKay, 2005).

Colleagues at the University of Pennsylvania and I are currently conducting a study that incorporates patient choice in the treatment protocol. Cocaine-dependent patients who fail to engage successfully in IOP are randomly assigned to one of two conditions that include motivational interviewing (MI) delivered by telephone. In one condition, the MI is directed toward resolving ambivalence regarding participating in IOP. In the other condition, patients are offered a choice of four possible treatment approaches, and the MI is used to help them select the best fit for them. These options are standard treatment at the IOP, individual cognitive–behavioral therapy (CBT) at a different setting (Carroll, 1998), a telephone-based stepped-care approach (McKay, Lynch, Shepard, & Pettinati, 2005), and a medical approach that combines the medication modafinil plus brief medication management sessions (Dackis et al., 2005). Patients who initially engage in IOP but drop out subsequently are also randomized to two conditions that both include MI. Once again, one condition involves MI focused on reengagement in IOP, whereas the other uses MI to help patients select from one of the same four treatment approaches. Although prior studies in the addictions have followed people who selected a particular treatment option (McKay et al., 1998; Weisner et al., 2000; Witbrodt et al., 2007), this is one of the first studies in the addictions to have evaluated the impact of providing patients with a range of treatment options.

One important ethical issue raised by offering choice of treatments to patients is the possible consequences of including lower intensity interventions. On the one hand, there is the concern that patients already having trouble at a higher level of treatment intensity will do even worse with lower intensity treatment, or with a treatment that does not stress abstinence. On the other hand, it is possible that some participation in a low-intensity intervention is better in the long run than no participation in a more intensive intervention.

Provide Incentives

The second approach to increasing rates of compliance with treatment modifications in adaptive protocols is to provide incentives of some sort. Studies have consistently shown that one type of incentive, contingency management (CM), improves drug use outcomes (Higgins et al., 2003; Petry, 2000; Silverman, Robles, Mudric, Bigelow, & Stitzer, 2004), and several studies have found that providing incentives for attendance increases retention in substance abusers (Brooner et al., 2004; Helmus, Saules, Schoener, & Roll, 2003; Rhodes et al., 2003; Svikis et al., 1997). In these studies, patients "earn" incentives in the form of vouchers that can be exchanged for goods and services consistent with a prorecovery lifestyle. The studies described in chapter 4 provided strong evidence that low-level incentives can help improve rates of participation in continuing care.

Persistence and Advance Directives

Maintaining good contact with patients in disease management protocols sometimes falls to persistent efforts on the part of the therapist or researcher. Dr. Chris Scott and colleagues at Chestnut Health Systems have developed procedures to maintain extremely high follow-up rates over periods of several years or more (Scott, 2004). These procedures include attention to patient education and motivation at the beginning of the protocol, collection of extensive and verified locator information, between-assessment contacts by mail and telephone, confirmation of follow-up appointments before the follow-up date, standardized tracking procedures, and frequent case review meetings. Although some of Scott's procedures are practical only in the context of a research study, the take-home message is that keeping in contact with patients is a function of work at the beginning of treatment (e.g., verified locator contacts) and obsessive efforts later on.

One technique that we use in our studies is to talk directly with patients at the beginning of the protocol about what to do if we lose track of them later on. This technique has been referred to as *advanced directives*, because it involves getting the patient's suggestions of actions that might be taken to help him or her if treatment does not go well and obtaining permission to try these actions. Our questions are focused around two issues:

1. What are the warning signals or red flags that indicate you are likely to stop participating in continuing care?
2. How will we be able to reach you if you stop contacting us?

After gathering this information, we ask patients for permission to call their attention to red flags if they occur later on and to bring up the potential implications of these warning signals. We also ask what might persuade them to get back in touch with us if they stop participating and do not return telephone calls. Because patients are often more motivated for treatment at the beginning, we find that they are willing to discuss these issues and usually make a real effort to give us the kind of information that might help us find and reengage them at a later date.

LACK OF VIABLE TREATMENT ALTERNATIVES

In depression and certain medical disorders such as cancer or hypertension, there are a number of effective medications and, in some cases, effective behavioral interventions. In addition, effective medications are available with different mechanisms of action. The availability of a menu of effective medications or behavioral treatments with different mechanisms of action greatly facilitates the development of adaptive treatment algorithms, because it increases the possibility that the second or third steps of the treatment algorithm will be effective with patients who do not respond to the first step. This is because subsequent steps that consist of interventions with different mechanisms of action can be selected. Conversely, if the second-step treatment is really not that different from the first step, it is less likely that nonresponders to the first step will become responders at the second step.

Medication Options

In contrast, with the addictions we currently have a fairly limited menu of effective medications to choose from, as was discussed in chapter 10. As noted earlier, there are three Food and Drug Administration–approved medications for alcoholism at this point. Fortunately, a number of other medications in the research pipeline that have shown promise, including topiramate and ondansetron (Johnson et al., 2000, 2007). These new agents have different mechanisms of action than the three currently approved alcohol medications and should therefore make possible a fuller menu of pharmacological choices for adaptive algorithms.

Psychotherapeutic Treatment Options

There is also some question about how truly different various psychotherapeutic interventions are from one another with regard to mechanisms of therapeutic action. One school of thought is that general factors such as empathy, positive regard for the patient, the therapeutic alliance, and the experience of talking openly with a caring person about one's problems explain much of the effect of talk-based interventions, whether they be behavioral, cognitive, psychodynamic, or motivational in focus (Wampold, 2001). Other theorists assert that although general factors are important, specific factors also make significant contributions to the determination of therapeutic outcomes (DeRubeis, Brotman, & Gibbons, 2005). In the addictions, specific factors include increases in motivation, improvements in social skills such as drink refusal, attendance at 12-step meetings, and so forth. As noted earlier, however, studies in the addictions that have addressed the issue of identifying the active ingredients, or mediators, of treatment effects have generally failed to confirm the importance of specific therapeutic factors in accounting for change, with the exception of self-help participation (Litt, Kadden, Kabela-Cormier, & Petry, 2003; Longabaugh, Wirtz, Beattie, Noel & Stout, 1995; Morgenstern & Longabaugh, 2000; Morgenstern & McKay, 2007; Tonigan, Connors, & Miller, 2003).

One approach that has been used in psychotherapy research to investigate the relative effect of general versus specific factors is meta-analysis. Baskin, Tierney, Minami, and Wampold (2003) hypothesized that if specific factors were accounting for treatment effects, studies that compared treatments such as CBT with purported specific therapeutic factors to generic treatments that featured general therapeutic factors only would yield significant differences favoring the treatments with specific effects when combined in meta-analyses. The results of the meta-analysis indicated that the treatments with specific factors were in fact not superior to comparison conditions that featured a similar "dose" of general factors.

Another meta-analysis included 80 outcomes studies that each contained a no-treatment control condition, a generic common factors condition, and an active treatment condition with specific factors (Stevens, Hynan, & Allen, 2000). Here, the results indicated that the common factors treatments were superior to placebo, and the specific factors treatments were superior to the common factors treatments. However, it should be noted that the common factors treatments in many of the studies were relatively weak interventions and probably contained fewer common or general therapeutic factors than the specific factors treatments. In any event, the key question for adaptive treatments is whether there is any reason to think that one behavioral intervention might succeed where another one had failed. It is probably safe to say that one has a greater chance of turning a nonresponder into a responder if the second treatment offered is clearly different from the first on at least one and probably two or more important dimensions, such as intensity, mode of delivery, purported mechanisms of action, and so forth.

GROUP RESULTS AND INDIVIDUALIZED TREATMENT

Ultimately, the goal of an adaptive treatment algorithm is to turn all patients into sustained responders by altering treatment to maximize response in all phases of care. This is truly patient-centered care because it is intended to result in treatment that is tailored expressly for each individual patient. However, there is a basic tension between the goal of individualized treatment and the methods used to achieve that goal (i.e., develop the adaptive algorithm)—at least when experimental methods are used to develop the algorithm.

The following example illustrates this issue. An alcohol treatment researcher wants to develop an optimal algorithm for outpatient treatment. One question that needs to be addressed is what to do with patients who drop out before becoming engaged in treatment. Because the investigator is not sure what approach might be best, she decides to randomly assign all early dropouts to one of three conditions: a treatment-as-usual (TAU) control, MI delivered by telephone, or a family-based intervention designed to leverage the patient back into treatment (FB). The latter two options were selected on the basis of prior research suggesting that they might be effective in reengaging early dropouts. The study results indicate that the family-based intervention produces statistically higher rates of reengagement in treatment and more abstinence days over the subsequent 3 months than either of the other two conditions. Therefore, the investigator concludes that the best adaptive algorithm is to give patients who drop out early a family intervention.

The problem with this conclusion is that despite these main effect results, some of the early dropouts do not do better in FB than MI or TAU. In fact, some of these patients actually did better in MI than FB. Anyone who has looked at data from a typical randomized clinical trial in the addictions no doubt has observed the large variation in individual scores around the group means. In an effort to use rigorous experimental methods to develop an optimal individualized treatment algorithm, the investigator is still relying on group averages rather than individual performance. One way to address this limitation is through additional randomizations for nonresponders. This was what was done in the STAR*D study of treatments for depression, described in chapter 7 of this volume. In that study, nonresponders were randomized multiple times, until they became responders (or reached the end of the protocol).

In our example, therefore, an ideal algorithm would have several steps, with the "best shot" treatment at each step decided by randomization:

1. Early dropouts should be given family-based treatment for 4 weeks.
2. If they are not reengaged, they should receive MI for an additional 4 weeks.
3. If they are still not reengaged, they should be offered a medication combined with a behavioral intervention.
4. If they are still not reengaged, incentives for participation should be added.

With multiple steps, each treatment decision can be based on what has worked best for the majority of patients, because the algorithm provides further directions on what to do next if what has worked best for the group is still not effective with a particular patient. The problem here is that conducting a study that will yield conclusive information (i.e., statistically significant results with all appropriate corrections to alpha levels) for three or four sequential decisions requires a very large sample size and a substantial budget. STAR*D, for example, involved almost 1,500 patients who did not respond to an initial trial of a standard antidepressant. At this point, it is probably premature to conduct a very-large-scale study with multiple sequential randomizations in the addictions because of limited National Institutes of Health budgets, relative paucity of viable therapeutic alternatives, and lack of interest and financial support from the pharmaceutical industry. If that is the case, how can the field of adaptive treatment move forward?

One possible solution is for the field to continue to focus on studies with up to two main randomizations that are powered sufficiently to find moderate-sized effects for those comparisons. This means sample sizes of between 250 and 350, depending on the number of conditions to which participants will be randomized and the outcome measures selected. These studies could also include a third randomization that would explore potential treatment options for participants who have still not responded to interventions provided earlier in the protocol. For example, patients who still are not responding after two stages in the protocol could be randomized either to continue to receive their Stage 2 treatment plus some augmentation or to receive the Stage 2 treatment alone. If the augmentation appears to improve outcomes for those patients on the basis of effect size comparisons rather than statistical significance, this apparent effect could be subjected to a replication test in a subsequent, adequately powered study.

TIMING OF THE ASSESSMENT OF TAILORING VARIABLES

As discussed in chapter 6, one of the key components of an adaptive treatment algorithm is the tailoring variable, or variables. Tailoring variables are closely monitored over time, and changes on these variables trigger changes in the treatment protocol, according to the rules of the algorithm. One important issue in the design of an adaptive continuing care intervention is how often the tailoring variable should be assessed. This decision is affected by several factors, including the goal of the intervention, available resources, and patient burden. For example, the goal of the recovery management checkups protocol developed by Scott and Dennis (2002) is to find former patients, assess their recent substance use, and link to treatment those who have been using heavily. Therefore, the primary point of the intervention is to keep slips from developing into more major relapses or to end relapses that have already happened, rather than prevent any episodes of use per se. For this goal, assessment every 3 months seems reasonable.

In contrast, adaptive protocols that attempt to prevent relapses would need to assess tailoring variables at much more frequent intervals. For example, the work of Shiffman and Waters (2004), described in chapter 2, suggests that increases in bad mood over the span of periods as short as a few hours predict relapse to smoking. Obviously, even well-funded research studies usually do not have the resources to assess patients several times a day, and most patients would probably not agree to such an assessment schedule even if it were feasible to provide it. In most cases, the assessment of tailoring variables is more likely to occur at weekly or monthly intervals. Because of this, it can be important to urge patients to call in between regularly scheduled sessions if their status suddenly worsens, so that there will be a chance to modify their treatment before more damage is done.

EVALUATING ADAPTIVE PROTOCOLS

As has been discussed in earlier chapters, there are two basic types of adaptive treatment studies: one in which randomization is used to develop the treatment algorithm and one in which a developed adaptive treatment algorithm is compared against another treatment condition. Each type of study presents certain challenges and issues in planning and conducting data analyses and in the interpretation of results. This section examines and discusses research designs and statistical approaches for building adaptive interventions, analyses used to compare adaptive interventions with other treatment conditions, identification of key treatment process variables, evaluation of the impact of providing patients with choice in treatment, and statistical power.

Analyses in an Adaptive Treatment Study Design

In the experimental approach, which is also referred to as an *adaptive treatment study design*, randomization is used to determine some or all of the following: cutting scores on tailoring measures, intervention options, and decision rules. Of course, it is not possible to experimentally manipulate more than a few of these factors, unless a very large sample size is available. However, to develop a full algorithm, it is usually necessary to conduct more than one randomization per subject. An adaptive study that includes multiple randomizations has been referred to as a *sequential multiple assignment randomized trial* (SMART) by Murphy, Lynch, McKay, Oslin, and Ten Have (2007). In the Oslin project described in chapter 9, for example, the first randomization is to two definitions of *nonresponse*. The second randomization is done separately within responder and nonresponder arms and involves comparisons of two continuing care strategies within each arm. This study design produces eight separate treatment algorithms, all of which could theoretically be compared against each other. Obviously, this situation is much more complicated than a simple two group comparison between an adaptive protocol and a control condition.

The key concept in analyzing a SMART study is that the analyses concern the comparison of algorithms or strategies, rather than specific treatments or treatment components. The same treatment component—for example, CBT or MI—could be present in more than one of the algorithms. In the Oslin study, all eight of the treatment algorithms include step up to a CBT-type treatment (i.e., combined behavioral intervention) for nonresponders, and four of the eight include continuation of naltrexone for nonresponders. The analyses are not designed to study any of these components in isolation or without consideration of other possible effects. So the relevant question is not simply whether continuing naltrexone will help initial nonresponders. Rather, what the analyses are really focusing on is identifying the combination of decision rules and interventions that produces the best outcome, however that is defined.

The fact that the analyses are comparing algorithms raises interesting questions about the selection of outcomes on which to focus. One could make the case that measures of key symptoms (e.g., days of heavy drinking, days of cocaine use) assessed during the adaptive protocol and over some posttreatment follow-up period would be the best outcome on which to focus. However, because the goal of the algorithm is essentially to make all patients responders, even if it takes a few treatment modifications, it might make more sense to assess symptoms or status toward the end of the treatment period, after each component of the algorithm has had an opportunity to exert an effect. In that case, the outcome might be heavy drinking days in the last 4 weeks of a 16-week algorithm or something to that effect. In the case of continuing care, however, in which interventions are likely to extend over longer periods of time, it is important to consider outcomes over the entire period, not just at the end of the intervention or follow-up. This is because the goal of continuing care is to maintain good outcomes, with greater success associated with more prolonged periods of symptom remission.

Comparing an Adaptive Algorithm With Treatment as Usual

The most straightforward—and familiar—study design for many in the field is the randomized two-group comparison, in which participants are randomly assigned to an experimental or control condition and followed for some period of time. This basic design can be used to evaluate the efficacy or effectiveness of an adaptive protocol versus TAU or some other control condition. The main difference is that in the case of the adaptive treatment condition, different participants are getting different combinations of treatments, whereas in the control condition, everyone is getting pretty much the same thing. That is, patients in the adaptive condition may be getting stepped up to higher intensity treatments, or switching to lower intensity treatments, or getting their basic treatment augmented with other interventions. The main effect analyses will be able to determine whether this package or algorithm works better than the comparison condition, but they will not shed any light on which aspects of the algorithm were particularly effective—or not effective. For example, the efficacy of an adaptive treatment algorithm might stem largely from providing more treatment to nonresponders, or conversely it might be due to providing ambivalent participants with less intensive alternatives.

Short-Term Follow-Ups in the Context of Extended Continuing Care

At this point, most studies of psychosocial or behavioral treatments for addiction feature follow-ups that extend beyond the end of treatment for at least 3 months, and often for as long as a year or more. Studies with longer posttreatment follow-up periods tend to be seen as stronger than those with shorter follow-ups because it is desirable to be able to show that treatment effects persist for extended periods after the intervention has ended. The major exception to this general trend has been pharmacotherapy trials, which are often only 8 to 12 weeks in length and do not typically follow patients beyond the end of period in which medications are provided. However, it should be noted that even pharmacotherapy trials occasionally feature longer term, postmedication follow-ups (Anton et al., 2006).

Although the goal of any adaptive continuing care intervention is good long-term outcomes, the primary focus is on the short-term impact of treatment modifications. Consider an algorithm that randomly assigns alcohol patients who do not show a good response to standard 12-step-based group treatment to either an augmentation condition (e.g., add MI) or a switch condition (e.g., drop standard treatment and provide a combination of naltrexone and medication management). The most pressing question is which of these two modifications turns a higher percentage of the nonresponders into responders—relatively quickly, before further deterioration and likely dropout occur. Therefore, the most appropriate follow-up period is probably 1 to 2 months, not 6 or 12 months.

This suggests that when developing an adaptive algorithm through experimental procedures, an investigator should concentrate on short evaluation periods after each randomization. In addition to focusing on the most critical period, this approach also has the advantage of producing shorter and consequently less expensive studies. In a given 5-year period, for example, an investigator could conduct a number of tests of various options at decision points in an adaptive algorithm, which is particularly advantageous if the first or second treatment options selected for examination prove less effective in turning nonresponders into responders than was expected. In addition, the brief evaluation periods also facilitate the implementation of sequential randomization trials.

After the tailoring variables, decision rules, and treatment alternatives that produce the highest rates of short-term response are selected, the resulting package can be tested against a comparison condition in a standard randomized controlled trial. In this confirmatory study, a longer term follow-up can, and probably should, be used to indicate how durable outcomes are in the group that receives the adaptive package, relative to outcomes in those who receive TAU.

Assessment of Mediation Effects

As was discussed in earlier chapters, there is considerable interest among addiction behavioral treatment researchers in trying to understand mechanisms of change within empirically supported interventions. The gold standard for the process of identifying mechanisms of action involves applying the set of analyses described by Baron and Kenny (1986), or updated versions of these analyses as described by McKinnon and Lockwood (2003), to data from randomized studies. Essentially, the treatment researcher is trying to (a) find an effect of the intervention on a key treatment process variable that theoretically should be affected by the intervention; (b) determine whether that process measure predicts subsequent outcome; and (c) test whether the treatment effect is accounted for, or mediated, by that process variable.

In an adaptive treatment protocol, one can apply this approach to identify mediation effects. The potential problem is that adaptive treatments are not fixed; rather, they are modified over time on the basis of patient performance. This means that the tailoring variable cannot also be a mediation variable, at least in the classic sense. An example may help to illustrate this. An investigator designs an adaptive treatment intervention, in which changes in self-efficacy serve as the tailoring variable. If self-efficacy goes up and stays up for at least 4 weeks, the intensity of the intervention is reduced. However, if self-efficacy drops by more than 20%, the intervention is augmented by more intensive approaches to raise coping skills and improve responses in high-risk situations.

Our investigator also believes that the impact of his adaptive intervention will be mediated by changes in self-efficacy, on the basis of the theory that was used to construct the intervention. The problem is that there is no longer a simple relation between self-efficacy and outcome. Patients in the adaptive condition who have low self-efficacy will get additional interventions, which will hopefully improve their outcome. So both high and low self-efficacy could be associated with good outcomes. Consequently, there may be no significant relation between within-treatment self-efficacy and outcome in this intervention. One solution to this problem is to eliminate the tailoring variable(s) from the search for possible mediating variables.

Evaluating Interventions That Feature Patient Choice

Adaptive interventions do not have to include patient choice with regard to treatment options. However, for interventions that do include this feature, there are additional analytic considerations. Perhaps the first issue is whether the relative effectiveness of the treatments that patients select can be compared in any way. For example, if a study gives patients the option of face-to-face or telephone continuing care, can outcomes in these two approaches be compared? The main problem is the potential effect of self-selection bias; in other words, the people who chose each of these two options may differ on many important factors other than preference for one of the modalities—factors that could influence outcome. Propensity scores or some other statistical method could be used to try to control for such differences, but the bottom line is the comparison might still be biased, and the results will therefore not be as persuasive as those obtained in a randomized comparison. However, from the perspective of adaptive treatments, more important questions might concern how many patients select each of the treatment options offered and whether the complete package yields better outcomes than an intervention that does not provide choice or one that provides a different menu of options.

A second consideration is power to detect significant effects and consequent sample size requirements. A research design that fully isolates and tests the overall effect of choice and the relative effectiveness of each therapeutic option would involve randomly assigning participants to one condition in which they are rerandomized to one of several treatments versus another condition in which they are allowed to select from the same set of treatments. In this study, one main analysis would compare the choice versus no-choice overall conditions, whereas subsequent analyses could compare treatment group effects in the no-choice condition (randomization; high level of causal inference possible) and the choice condition (no randomization; low level of causal inference possible). To address both of these questions, the study would need to be powered to find differences between the treatment groups in the no-choice condition.

CONCLUSION

The field of adaptive treatment is still in its relative infancy, and a number of issues and challenges in implementation and evaluation need further attention. In this chapter, I have considered problems with retention and compliance, the need for more viable behavioral and pharmacological treatment options, the tension between what is best for the "average" patient and the therapeutic needs of individuals, the optimal timing of the assessment of tailoring variables, implications of considering patient preference, various data-analytic concerns, and statistical power. Some of these challenges are common to all continuing care interventions for substance use disorders, whereas others are more specific to adaptive treatment—or at least potentially more important.

The good news is that innovative clinicians and researchers are making notable headway with many of these problems. More effective ways of keeping patients engaged in treatment are available, and the range of effective interventions to choose from keeps expanding. Moreover, thanks to the work of Susan Murphy and other statisticians, there have been considerable improvements in procedures to evaluate adaptive interventions and determine appropriate sample sizes for research studies. That said, one of the major challenges that remains is how to deliver modifications to patients who are not doing well and are in the process of pulling away from treatment. One could argue that these are the patients who are most in need of some sort of change to the treatment they are getting and least likely to be receptive to any continued involvement in treatment, no matter how it is modified. This is likely to be a major focus of research efforts in the coming years.

Part IV of this book has provided a close look at several current adaptive treatment studies that have included continuing care phases, information on how to develop and implement adaptive continuing care protocols, and a review of some of the challenges likely to be encountered in designing and implementing these protocols. In Part V, other novel approaches to continuing care and disease management for substance use disorders are described, a final summary of key points is provided, and closing thoughts about where the field of continuing care is likely to go are offered.

V

NEW DEVELOPMENTS AND FUTURE DIRECTIONS

12

OTHER DEVELOPMENTS IN DISEASE MANAGEMENT FOR SUBSTANCE USE DISORDERS

In earlier chapters, a number of fixed and adaptive continuing care models were presented and reviewed, and research on these models was described. There are other exciting developments in extended care for addiction, which are described in this chapter. These include newer case management approaches, intensive recovery coaching, alternative service delivery settings, integrated care models, linkage to community supports, and recovery-based approaches. In addition, recent innovations in technology have considerably expanded the potential for major advances in how patients are monitored over time and in how treatment is delivered.

One important commonality across these new models is that many address most of the primary goals of the chronic care model, as described by Wagner et al. (2001). These goals include support for patient self-management, links to community resources, interventions to increase self-confidence and skill levels, a focus on goal setting, and identification of barriers to achieving goals and methods to overcome such barriers. The Institute of Medicine (IOM) has also strongly recommended that treatment facilities—including those treating alcohol and drug use disorders (see IOM, 2001, 2006)— provide care that is *patient-centered*. Patient-centered care is expected, among other things, to be attractive, responsive to the needs of patients, and respectful of their rights to know all available options for the treatment of their condition (IOM, 2006).

CASE MANAGEMENT FOR HIGH-COST PATIENTS

Virtually all the continuing care interventions described in this book have been intended for all patients in a particular treatment program or research study—at least those who meet inclusion criteria for the study. The assumption underlying this approach is that all patients with substance use disorders who end up in the formal treatment system could benefit from continuing care. However, in many other disorders, disease management interventions are targeted to particular individuals who are the most difficult and expensive to manage. These approaches are driven by the commonly observed fact that a relatively small group of patients account for the lion's share of costs in the medical system—"20% of the patients account for 80% of the costs" is one statistic that is often quoted. Such programs are adaptive, in that patient-cost data serve as a tailoring variable that triggers entry into the disease management protocol when costs exceed an established threshold.

The Indiana Chronic Disease Management Program is an example of an innovative attempt to improve care and lower costs of managing Medicaid members with chronic disorders such as congestive heart failure, diabetes, and asthma (Rosenman et al., 2006). In this program, potentially eligible participants are identified to create regional registries. A risk stratification algorithm was developed that considered total net Medicaid claims costs in the prior year, Medicaid aid category, and total number of unique medications filled in the past year. Using this algorithm, participants were placed in one of three categories: most costly 20%, next most costly 30%, and lowest cost 50%.

Nurse care managers were assigned to the most costly 20% of participants. In home visits, the nurses provided education to patients and family, encouraged self-management, facilitated communication with physicians, and made referrals to community resources. Telephone follow-up was provided between home visits. The rest of the participants (the lower 80%, as determined by cost) were provided with care management by telephone only. A Web-based information system was used to coordinate care, provide decision support, and enter and retrieve care plans and progress notes. Finally, medical practices involved with the program were invited to participate in quality improvement collaboratives. The practices in these collaboratives set quality improvement goals, reported on progress, and shared ideas through e-mail and conference calls.

In the field of addiction treatment, several new programs are attempting to manage expensive patients with more intensive monitoring and case management. Starting in September 2006, New York state began to implement a $25 million disease management program for high utilizers of Medicaid services in 23 counties. This effort is led by the single state substance abuse agency: the Office of Alcoholism and Substance Abuse Services (OASAS). This new program, titled Managed Addiction Treatment Services (MATS), has provided counties with funding to develop case management program that outreach, engage, assess, monitor, and link patients to needed care across substance abuse, mental health, medical, and social service systems.

In this program, OASAS provides the county each month with a list of names of individuals who have incurred costs above a threshold (> $10,000). These individuals are deemed "MATS Eligible" and receive case management services for up to 1 year. An attractive feature of MATS is that the effort is located and led at the county level, at which medical, behavioral health, and social services are coordinated. In addition, county government bears a share of the financial costs for high-cost patients and therefore has a direct and immediate monetary incentive to coordinate and improve care. The goal of the intervention is to get patients engaged in appropriate levels of care across different systems and to reduce Medicaid costs due to inappropriate or inefficient use of high-cost crisis services (e.g., inpatient care, emergency department). OASAS collects administrative data on performance measures such as rates of engagement in case management as well as service utilization and cost of crisis services.

These disease management interventions for expensive patients can actually be seen as a form of adaptive treatment. The tailoring variable is something like total treatment costs in the prior year, number of detoxifications not followed by rehabilitation, or some other objective measure of drain on the system. Cutting scores on the tailoring variables are established, and when a patient exceeds that score, transition into the disease management program is triggered. By following such adaptive procedures, the interventions are directed at those who probably most need extended care—patients who fail to complete treatment and consequently require expensive detoxification and emergency department care. It is worth noting that standard aftercare procedures, as described in chapter 3, have typically been offered only to patients who complete their initial level of care (e.g., residential treatment, intensive outpatient program). These patients may in fact be the ones who will least benefit from continuing care because they have had a good initial response to treatment. Meanwhile, the patients most in need of continuing care are guaranteed not to receive it.

INTENSIVE RECOVERY COACHING

Recovery coaches provide extended, and sometimes intensive, continuing care, often through a number of modalities (White, 2008). For example, recovery coaches may meet individually with the patients on a regular basis; are often available by telephone at all hours; may arrange for other services, such as psychiatric and medical care; may escort patients to self-help meetings and other prorecovery activities; and may arrange meetings with others in recovery. Some recovery coaches will also work with the patient's family in whatever way is most helpful to the patient's recovery, which might include negotiating conflicts and disagreements, arranging visits, or providing a conduit for information when direct contact between the patient and family is contraindicated for some reason.

At this point, there are many individuals and companies that provide intensive recovery coaching. One such company, Recovery Support Services, provides a comprehensive menu of services, linked by Web technology. Services are coordinated by a program monitor, who meets regularly with the patient by telephone, reviews biological fluid monitoring results (i.e., urine drug screens) and daily activity data submitted by the patient via the Internet, and keeps track of other factors such as 12-step attendance, education, community service, workplace behavior, and family functioning. Recovery Support Services is a strong advocate of transparency in recovery and open communication between people who are supporting the patient's recovery. To this end, the company uses an Internet-based system that immediately and automatically informs family members, addiction treatment providers, other health care providers, and other authorized individuals when a patient fails to complete a component of the program (R. Armstrong, personal communication, October 4, 2007).

The intensive recovery coach approach to continuing care has a number of obvious strengths, particularly as a follow-up to residential care. It provides highly individualized assistance "on the ground," so to speak, to patients as they reenter their communities. The flexibility of the services is in keeping with wide variations both between and within individuals with regard to need for services at various points in the recovery process. Frequent contacts allow for rapid detection of deteriorations in functioning and prorecovery behaviors, as well as any episodes of substance use.

However, the highly flexible and individualized nature of these interventions could also be a potential weakness. The recovery coaches or care managers are often free within relatively broad limits to deliver the intervention as they see fit, rather than follow a detailed treatment algorithm. Therefore, behaviors that might trigger a modification in the intensity of care in the case of one patient might not result in any change in another patient, particularly if that person is working with a different recovery coach or care manager. Also, it should be stressed that the effectiveness of these programs has not been evaluated in controlled studies.

ALTERNATIVE SERVICE DELIVERY SETTINGS

There is increasing recognition that many individuals with substance use disorders are not interested in or willing to participate in traditional, addiction specialty treatment programs. There are several reasons for this. Many people do not want to stop drinking entirely and therefore object to the total abstinence orientation of these programs. Others do not like other aspects of Alcoholics Anonymous (AA)–based treatment, including the focus on spiritual matters, use of group therapy, and the expectation of a major commitment of time (e.g., 90 meetings in 90 days). Finally, there can still be considerable stigma attached with "going to rehab," which sours many people on the idea of traditional treatment. Accurate estimates of the percentage of people with addiction who will not go into traditional treatment are not yet available, but research does show that only about 10% of those with substance use disorders get treatment in a given year (IOM, 2001, 2006). Some of this is due to lack of available treatment slots, but resistance to standard treatment models is also no doubt an important factor in the large percentage of untreated individuals.

One of the innovative approaches to addressing this problem has been the use of alternative service delivery systems to provide addiction care. One of the most promising of these efforts has been in primary medical care practices. Fleming, Barry, Manwell, Johnson, and London (1997) demonstrated that physicians could screen for alcohol use disorders in primary care and deliver effective brief interventions. Recently, protocols have been developed to provide more extended treatment of alcohol use disorders in primary care for patients who do not want or are otherwise not appropriate for treatment in traditional programs. For example, a model referred to as *alcohol care management* is being used in some Veterans Affairs Medical Centers (VAMC), and has been described in the Veterans Affairs Practice Guidelines. Under this model, patients are followed in primary care, and addiction-focused pharmacotherapy is discussed and implemented if acceptable to the patient. At subsequent visits, substance use is monitored and encouragement for reductions in use or abstinence is provided, along with motivational support. Participation in self-help groups is recommended, any nicotine use is addressed, and help for social, financial, and housing problems is provided or referrals are made. Patients who do not achieve stabilization under this approach are given a referral to specialty care.

At the Philadelphia VAMC, Oslin et al. (2006) developed a telephone-based service delivery system, called the Behavioral Health Lab (BHL), which is integrated with primary care practices through the Web. The BHL was created as a service to primary care providers for assessing and managing mental health and substance abuse problems. It assists in the evaluation of patients who are identified by screening or clinical assessment and can assist in the management of an array of problems, including substance misuse, depression, or anxiety. The BHL functions much like a clinical chemistry laboratory in that it conducts structured assessments with patient information that is entered directly into a computer software program. The program provides decision support allowing for the determination of the appropriate level of clinical service and prompts the staff to conduct assessments at several predetermined follow-ups. BHL staff work with each provider to develop treatment plans or to get the patient to the appropriate care setting. In addition to the initial evaluation and triage function, the BHL can provide a number of additional services:

- brief interventions for excessive alcohol use or abuse;
- care management for depression or anxiety that provides monitoring for treatment response, adherence, and adverse effects for patients who are newly started on antidepressants, along with decision support for their providers;
- referral care for more complex cases needing specialty care services; and
- watchful waiting for patients with minor or subsyndromal depression, monitored weekly for up to 8 weeks, with treatment referral only if their symptoms persist or worsen, or if the veteran requests care.

Because several of the BHL components are telephone-based, the BHL can be delivered from a central location to any primary care practice, including remote sites. The software program, training manuals, and algorithms can also be used in conjunction with existing staff who are already integrated into the primary care setting. The BHL has been implemented in more than 20 primary care clinics, with more than 6,500 patients assessed in the past 2 years (D. Oslin, personal communication, June 15, 2008). The BHL is also now being used by Blue Cross/Blue Shield of South Carolina.

There have been other efforts to integrate addiction treatment with either primary care or mental health treatment to promote higher rates of sustained participation in treatment. Weisner, Mertens, Parthasarathy, Moore, and Lu (2001) evaluated the effectiveness of locating primary health care within the addiction treatment program in an HMO, relative to the treatment-as-usual (TAU) model in which primary care and addiction treatment are entirely independent. For patients in this study with substance abuse–related medical conditions, the integrated model produced higher rates of abstinence at 6 months than TAU (69% vs. 55%, $p = .006$). A similar study by Saxon et al. (2006) randomized veterans entering substance use disorder treatment with a chronic medical condition and no current primary care to receive primary medical care either onsite in the VA substance use disorder clinic or in the VA general internal medicine clinic. The results indicated that patients receiving primary health care onsite were more likely to attend primary care appointments and to still be attending substance use disorder treatment at 3 months. However, there were no differences in substance use outcomes over a 12-month follow-up.

Samet et al. (2003) evaluated whether inpatient detoxification might be a point at which individuals who did not have a primary care physician could be linked to primary medical care. In the intervention, a multidisciplinary team conducted an initial evaluation at a detoxification program and provided facilitated referral and active linkage to an offsite primary care clinic. Participants in the study were randomized to this intervention or to a control condition. Results indicated that linkage to primary medical care occurred in 69% of the intervention group compared with 53% in the control group ($p = .0003$). The clinic was similarly effective for subjects with alcohol and illicit drug problems. Randomization to the active linkage condition resulted in no significant differences in secondary outcomes, which were addiction severity, health-related quality of life, use of medical and addiction services, and HIV risk behaviors. However, follow-up analyses by Saitz, Horton, Larson, Winter, and Samet (2005) indicated that patients who attended two or more primary care visits had lower odds of drug use or alcohol intoxication during follow-up.

COMMUNITY SUPPORTS

It has long been recognized that some individuals with substance use disorders have fallen out of normal patterns of functioning in society and are in need of help with housing, employment, and other basic life skills. The shift from residential to outpatient treatment has been particularly problematic for patients without stable, drug-free housing. In Philadelphia and other cities, this has led to the development of networks of *recovery houses*, which provide alcohol- and drug-free living situations for patients while they are in an intensive outpatient program and for some time afterward. Recovery houses are generally managed by peers who are further along in recovery, and many have some amount of recovery-oriented programming, which residents are required to attend. One of the limitations of many recovery houses, however, is that residents who relapse are not allowed to stay in the house.

William White has written extensively on the importance of the larger community as a potential resource for people in recovery (White, 1998, 2007, 2008, 2009). According to White, the goal of professional intervention should be to mobilize personal, family, and community resources to minimize the need for future professional assistance. White has recommended that recovery community building involve three steps: (a) extending professionally directed treatment services into the community, (b) better integrating community resources back into formal treatment programs, and (c) increasing the role of formal treatment in recovery advocacy and recovery community building efforts (White, 2009). A number of strategies that addiction counselors and programs can use to link patients in addiction treatment to sources of support in the community, described in a recent monograph by White and Kurtz (2006), are presented in Exhibit 12.1.

Litt et al. (2007) at the University of Connecticut, developed a treatment intervention designed to help patients change their social networks to become more supportive of abstinence. Because AA was the most readily available potential source of support for abstinence, the intervention made use of components from the 12-Step Facilitation Manual (Nowinski, Baker, & Carroll, 1995) developed for Project MATCH (Matching Alcohol Treatments to Client Heterogeneity). Making new acquaintances and engaging in enjoyable social activities at AA or other social networks were stressed, rather than other AA components such as the higher power and one's own powerlessness. For those participants who are not interested in AA, the intervention focused on increasing other forms of social support for abstinence.

This intervention, referred to as *network support* (NS), was then evaluated in a research study. Participants were randomized to a case management comparison condition (CM), NS, or NS plus incentives for abstinence (NS + ContM). Data from the 1-year follow-up indicated that both NS conditions produced better alcohol use outcomes than the case management intervention, as indicated by higher percent days abstinent (about 75% vs. 63%, $d = 0.41$) and higher rates of continuous abstinence in each 3-month period (as high as 40% in NS vs. 20% in CM). Moreover, NS led to greater increases in AA attendance and behavioral and attitudinal support for abstinence. It is interesting to note that the incentives did not improve outcome over NS alone—and in some cases, they actually appeared to decrease the effectiveness of NS. Further analyses of mechanisms of action indicated that the treatment worked by increasing social support for abstinence, not by decreasing social support for continued use (Litt, Kadden, Kabela-Cormier, & Petry, 2007).

RECOVERY-ORIENTED MODELS

The recovery movement combines elements of empowerment, self-help, self-determination, and civil rights. It was developed as an alternative to standard treatment for serious mental illnesses such as schizophrenia, for which there is no cure. The main goal of the recovery approach is to help people with these disorders lead full, productive, and socially connected lives

EXHIBIT 12.1
Strategies to Link Patients to Sources of Support in the Community

1. Educate each patient about the importance and potential benefits of posttreatment recovery support services.
2. Solicit each patient's past experiences with and perceptions (i.e., stereotypes) of recovery mutual-aid groups, and review the menu of posttreatment recovery support options (e.g., family, social, occupational, formal support groups).
3. Identify important meeting characteristics (e.g., religious, spiritual, secular; smoking or nonsmoking; gender; ethnicity; age; geographical access).
4. Use assertive rather than passive linkage procedures (e.g., orient each patient about what to expect in his or her first meeting).
5. Link each patient to a particular person to orient and guide the patient into a relationship with a local group, and link each patient to a specific meeting for his or her initial exposure.
6. Resolve obstacles to participation (e.g., day care, transportation).
7. Monitor and evaluate each patient's initial and ongoing responses to that person/meeting through follow-up phone calls, e-mails, or visits.
8. Link family members to support structures congruent with the recovery framework of the patient (e.g., referring spouses and children to Al-Anon and Alateen when the patient is participating in Alcoholics Anonymous).

Note. Data from White and Kurtz (2006).

(Davidson, O'Connell, Tondora, Lawless, & Evans, 2005). Proponents of the recovery model assert that there is no reason people with serious mental illness should not be able to participate fully in society, provided that they receive necessary supports.

The recovery model places greater emphasis on patient self-determination, particularly with regard to the setting of therapeutic goals and selection of treatments, than other psychiatric treatment approaches. The model stresses that those with psychiatric disorders want to be productive members of society, to feel that they "belong," and to be able to give back by helping others. The role of the therapist in a recovery model shifts from a focus on ameliorating symptoms and fixing problems to one of identifying, nurturing, and building strengths, talents, and interests. Similar to addiction treatment, the recovery model makes extensive use of peers to provide ongoing recovery support.

As described by Davidson et al. (2005), the common elements of recovery-oriented models are as follows:

- renewing hope and commitment,
- redefining the self,
- being involved in meaningful activities,
- overcoming stigma,
- assuming control,
- becoming empowered and exercising citizenship,
- managing symptoms, and
- being supported by others.

It is clear from these elements that the recovery movement has much in common with AA and other 12-step programs in addiction. However, there is more of a focus on the patient assuming control and being able to choose treatment goals and the methods to reach those goals. This is at odds, to some degree, with the emphasis in 12-step programs of turning one's will over to a higher power, as exemplified by the first step and slogans such as "getting out of the driver's seat."

The state of Connecticut has been engaged in active efforts since 1999 to shift its publicly funded mental health and substance use disorder treatment system to more of a recovery model. These efforts are described in *Practice Guidelines for Recovery-Oriented Behavioral Health Care*, published by the Connecticut Department of Mental Health and Addictions Services in 2006. Several portions of this document outline recovery-focused approaches to topics such as continuity of care, strengths-based assessment, individualized recovery planning, and identifying and addressing barriers to recovery. Some of the guiding principles include the following:

1. People should have a flexible array of options from which to choose.
2. Individuals are not expected or required to progress through a continuum of care in a linear or sequential manner.
3. Focus of care is on enhancing existing strengths and recovery capital. This means less focus on relapse prevention and more on the promotion of recovery.
4. Goals of the recovery plan are defined by the person and involve pursuing a life in the community.
5. Interventions are aimed at assisting people gain autonomy, power, and connections with others.
6. The range of valued expertise is expanded beyond specialized clinical professionals to include contributions of multiple individuals and services in the community.
7. People are actively involved in all aspects of their care including treatment planning, assessment, goal setting, and evaluation.
8. New technologies (e.g., telemedicine, Web-based applications, self-help resources) are incorporated as service options.
9. Access to housing, employment, and other supports that make recovery sustainable are enhanced.

Connecticut has established several peer-staffed recovery centers, to provide ongoing support to individuals with substance use disorders. These centers provide a range of services, including weekly telephone support calls made by experienced volunteers to people relatively new in their recoveries. The Connecticut Department of Mental Health and Addiction services reported that during the period of 2005 to 2007, volunteers at one recovery center provided support calls to 879 individuals. More than 12,000 calls were attempted, with approximately 4,000 completed (Connecticut Department of Mental Health and Addiction Services, 2007). Although this rate of call completion is relatively low, participants did receive, on average, more than four calls, and the use of peers to provide the calls no doubt increased the benefit–cost ratio of the intervention.

The recovery model has a number of potential strengths, including its focus on the development of strengths, emphasis on empowerment and self-determination, and involvement of the community in the recovery process. One concern about the recovery model approach is whether it can work with patients who have many of the co-occurring problems and issues that put them at high risk of relapse, such as significant psychiatric problems and low motivation for change. It can be extremely difficult for treatment providers to work with patients when they have continued to use heavily and are not expressing much interest in being an active participant in treatment of any sort, even if offered a choice. However, it is also possible that poor initial response to treatment could be due to some degree to the perception that treatment is not going to provide anything desirable.

INCORPORATION OF NEW TECHNOLOGIES

Three areas in which new technologies have the potential to drive major changes in the management of addictive disorders are monitoring of status and symptoms over time, the use of the Internet, and computerized delivery of treatment services.

Monitoring

There is now a large body of evidence that monitoring use of alcohol and drugs can play an important role in recovery. Up until fairly recently, the state of the art in monitoring has been administration of questionnaires or interviews at every treatment session to assess substance use and related factors. Although this represents an improvement over less frequent monitoring, such data are still limited because they are self-report—and thus not always valid—and because periods of high risk may be experienced between treatment sessions when no monitoring is occurring.

Ecological momentary assessment (EMA) and interactive voice recording (IVR), discussed in chapters 2 and 5, respectively, address one of these limitations by providing more frequent assessments of symptoms and other factors—up to several times per day in the case of EMA (R. L. Collins, Kashdan, & Gollnisch, 2003; T. L. Simpson, Kivlahan, Bush, & McFall, 2005). The problem of valid assessment can likely be addressed in the not-too-distant future by newer monitoring technologies, which measure levels of alcohol and drugs in the system and either store or transmit that information to a server set up to receive such data.

Gustafson et al. (2005), at the University of Wisconsin, have proposed the use of "smart phones," which could be carried by individuals in recovery from substance use disorders. These phones could be equipped with numerous features that facilitate contact with information and social supports, including CHESS (i.e., The Comprehensive Health Enhancement Support System), developed and tested by the Center for Health Systems Research and Analysis at the University of Wisconsin. Software in such phones could also be used to contact identified sources of social support, using global positioning systems to select a person who is closest geographically to the patient's current location.

Internet

An Internet-based survey was conducted with 928 individuals who reported using Internet communication and support tools for prevention, intervention, recovery, or aftercare for alcohol, nicotine, or other substance use problems (M. J. Hall & Tidwell, 2003). The respondents reported that they had been using Internet recovery–related services for an average of 31 months. More than 55 Internet recovery plans or services were identified by the respondents. Therefore, it appears that a considerable number of Internet-based addiction treatment resources are currently available and in use by significant numbers of people with addiction-related concerns. Here, I briefly focus on one of the more comprehensive Internet continuing care programs.

Hazelden, one of the first of the 28-day Minnesota model AA-based treatment programs, has developed and implemented a highly innovative, adaptive, Web-based continuing care program. This program, called My Ongoing Recovery Experience (MORE), has been developed through a collaboration between Hazelden and HealthMedia, of Ann Arbor, Michigan. In its final form, MORE will provide up to 18 months of adaptive continuing care for patients who have received an initial phase of acute residential treatment at Hazelden. MORE consists of seven interactive modules that address various challenges in the recovery process, through the provision of monitoring and assessment, feedback, support, information, and suggestions for dealing with relapse risk factors. The modules are engaging and tailored to characteristics of the patient. Patients must complete each module before gaining access to subsequent modules, although they are free to return to completed modules at any time. The program also features a personal home page for each participant, progress checks, a journal, workbook activities, a calendar of key upcoming events, a library of recovery materials, and lists of Hazelden alumni contacts.

MORE also arranges for contact with counselors at Hazelden, through several mechanisms. First, counselors are prompted to contact a patient in their case load when a red flag is triggered, because of warning signs of relapse provided by the patient through MORE or by failure of a patient to use MORE for a given period of time. Second, patients can leave e-mail messages through MORE requesting telephone contact with a counselor. MORE qualified as an adaptive treatment protocol because it measures patient progress at regular intervals through standardized measures and provides explicit guidelines for modifying continuing care on the basis of performance. Overall, MORE is a promising package, by virtue of its high-quality and appealing visual presentation, breadth of content, interactive capabilities, adaptive nature, and ability to coordinate Web-based and counselor-provided services. The Department of Veterans Affairs is also working on a Web-based recovery support system for the use of veterans and their families that will ultimately have some of the same features as MORE.

Computerized Delivery of Treatment Services

Computers have been used to provide treatment or promote health behaviors for a variety of disorders, including Alzheimer's disease, arthritis, asthma, anxiety and depression, diabetes, heart disease, HIV, hypertension, smoking cessation, and cancer (Bickel & Marsch, 2007). Several recent studies have demonstrated that computers can deliver effective interventions for substance use disorders. One such example is the computer-based training for cognitive–behavioral therapy (CBT4CBT) program developed by Carroll et al. (2008), described in chapter 3 of this volume. This interactive program delivers a cognitive–behavioral intervention for substance use disorders and can be used as an adjunct to standard care.

Now there also is evidence that the community reinforcement approach (CRA) can be delivered effectively by computer. CRA is a complicated intervention that includes contingency management, problem solving, social skills training, anger management, relapse prevention, vocational counseling, drug-refusal training, social/recreational counseling, and a number of other components. Bickel, Marsch, Buchhalter, and Badger (2008) compared therapist-delivered CRA with vouchers, computer-assisted CRA with vouchers, and TAU in a sample of opiate-dependent patients who were receiving standard psychosocial treatment and buprenorphine. Results indicated that the two CRA conditions did not differ on weeks of continuous opiate and cocaine abstinence (mean of 8.0 vs. 7.8 weeks in therapist- and computer-delivered CRA, respectively). Both conditions did better than standard care (mean of 4.7 weeks of continuous abstinence). The good results that have been obtained with CBT4CBT and computer-assisted CRA will likely spur the development of other computer-assisted interventions for substance use disorders and lead to their wider adoption in the treatment system.

CONCLUSION

This chapter described a number of new models of extended care, including case management for high-cost patients, intensive recovery coaching, alternative service delivery settings, integrated care models, linkage to community supports, and recovery-based approaches. These models share a number of features, including individualized care, delivery of treatment outside of standard specialty clinics, and linkage of patients to community supports. The goals of these models are consistent with those of Wagner's chronic care model (Wagner et al., 2001) in that they strive for better patient self-management, greater linkage to community resources, identification of barriers to achieving goals and methods to overcome such barriers, better integrated care, and improved information technology. It should also be noted that there is at this point relatively little research on the effectiveness of these approaches.

The case management approaches discussed in this chapter are, by definition, adaptive, in that the selection of patients for these interventions is based on how much high-cost treatment has been received in the past year. In other words, patients receive case management if the cost of their addiction services in the past year (i.e., the tailoring variable) exceeds a certain threshold. Intensive recovery coaching can also be adaptive in that the patient's progress in recovery is used to determine the frequency, intensity, and nature of the recovery coach's interactions with the patient and significant others. However, recovery coaches appear to differ on how specific their adaptive algorithms are. For example, Recovery Support Services makes use of a Web-based system that automatically sends out alerts when patients are not compliant with their recovery program. Conversely, it is less clear to what extent other recovery coaches make use of specific algorithms in determining how to tailor their efforts to patient progress in recovery over time. Integrated care efforts are also tailored in that they are designed to facilitate better care for patients with addiction and co-occurring disorders.

Virtually all of these approaches involve the use of interventions that are delivered outside of standard specialty care clinics, where most continuing care has traditionally been delivered (see chap. 3). The Internet, telephone, recovery coaching, and intensive case management all involve bringing treatment to the patient's home or wherever he or she is currently living. Alternative service delivery approaches such as Oslin et al.'s (2006) BHL also involve telephone-based treatment delivery or delivery at other facilities such as primary care clinics or community mental health centers. Community support models and recovery-oriented models are focused on helping patients link to and engage with resources in the community that can provide assistance with important issues such as housing, education, child care, skill building, employment, and so forth.

We will no doubt see considerably more empirical research on these new extended treatment models in the coming years. However, at this point, there is little solid evidence of their effectiveness. One exception to this is in the area of integrated care models. Research by Weisner et al. (2001), Saxon et al. (2001), Samet et al. (2003), and Saitz et al. (2005) indicates that providing basic medical care as part of addiction treatment led to better outcomes than more traditional models, which did not feature integrated care. Integrated care models presented in other chapters of this book have also been effective (e.g., Willenbring & Olson, 1999). The work of Litt et al. (2007) on increasing patients' social support for abstinence has also yielded positive results in a randomized trial and appears to be a highly promising approach for increasing community support for recovery. The final chapter of this book provides a summary and integration of what can be concluded at this point from research on continuing care and adaptive treatment models, along with final thoughts about where the field is headed and challenges that need to be addressed.

13

SUMMARY OF KEY POINTS AND FUTURE DIRECTIONS

The goal of this book has been to examine the effectiveness of current methods for enhancing sustained recovery in individuals with substance use disorders, with a particular focus on newer, adaptive approaches to continuing care. To that end, this book has reviewed biopsychosocial factors that point toward the potential value of extended care, the characteristics of effective continuing care, methods for enhancing participation in continuing care, and a host of newer approaches to managing addiction over time. The principles of adaptive treatment have been described, and examples of adaptive treatment algorithms in mental health and addiction have been presented. For clinicians interested in developing adaptive interventions, three chapters presented detailed information on how to design, implement, evaluate, and improve an adaptive continuing care protocol. Moreover, an adaptive telephone-based continuing care protocol is included as an appendix. This final chapter offers a brief summary of the main findings of this book and a discussion of issues in continuing care that require further research. Thoughts about future directions for the field are also presented.

EVOLUTION OF THE CONCEPT OF CONTINUING CARE

In most of the studies reviewed in chapter 3, there was a clear demarcation between the initial phase of care, which was usually residential or inpatient treatment or some form of intensive outpatient treatment, and continuing care. However, the field of addiction treatment is rapidly moving toward service delivery systems in which there is much less emphasis on transitioning between discrete levels of care. For example, much of the treatment in publicly funded programs is provided in longer term outpatient programs, where patients may move from an intensive outpatient program (IOP) to an outpatient (OP) program as they progress in treatment but remain in the same facility. Other examples of the move away from discrete levels of care are interventions in which patients with substance use disorders and other medical or psychiatric problems are managed in primary care or other medical settings where they can receive integrated care over time.

These changes in service delivery systems have and will continue to drive the evolution of continuing care models. It is now clear that patients should become engaged in continuing care early in the treatment process to help prevent early dropout and increase the likelihood of sustained engagement in care. Waiting to initiate continuing care until after patients have graduated from their first level of treatment has become problematic because many patients dropout rather than complete IOP or OP (M. D. Godley, Garner, Funk, Passetti, & Godley, 2008). Continuing care of all types is now seen as serving a disease management role in that brief therapeutic contacts and even extended monitoring can help facilitate patient self-care and connections with communities of recovery. Moreover, these contacts also provide an early-warning system that can facilitate reentry into more intensive forms of treatment when necessary (Dennis, Scott, & Funk, 2003). We may get to a point where continuing care as we know it now will really not exist as a separate phase of care but rather will be subsumed into continuing care–oriented service delivery systems. In such a system, patients who are diagnosed with chronic forms of substance use disorders (i.e., those who have had trouble with repeated relapses) will routinely receive extended care and monitoring as part of their service package.

WHAT DO WE KNOW ABOUT EFFECTIVE CONTINUING CARE?

Although the field of continuing care research is relatively new and still underresearched, the studies reviewed in this book tell a fairly consistent story about the factors that seem to be associated with more effective disease management. These factors include longer interventions, active efforts to reach and retain patients, use of incentives, and linkage to other sources of support in the community. Conversely, the specific orientation of the treatment and its intensity may be of less importance in determining effectiveness.

Duration Appears to Matter

In the reviews of continuing care studies in chapters 3, 5, and 8, interventions that featured longer treatment durations consistently demonstrated better outcomes over comparison conditions. Examples of these longer interventions included 12 months of behavioral marital therapy (O'Farrell, Choquette, & Cutter, 1998), home visits from a nurse provided over 12 months (Patterson, MacPherson, & Brady, 1997), telephone contact provided over 12 months or more (Foote & Erfurt, 1991; McKay, Lynch, Van Horn, et al., 2009), recovery checkups delivered quarterly over 24 months (Dennis et al., 2003), extended contingency management interventions (Silverman et al., 2002; Silverman, Robles, Mudric, Bigelow, & Stitzer, 2004), 12-month case management (Morgenstern et al., 2006), extended monitoring in primary care (Kristenson, Osterling, Nilsson, & Lindgarde, 2002), and extended integrated treatment models (Willenbring & Olson, 1999). These findings suggest that interventions with longer planned durations may have a greater likelihood of producing positive effects, as long as they also facilitate sustained engagement. However, additional studies are needed that directly compare short (e.g., 3-month) versus extended (e.g., 18-month) versions of the same intervention to determine if longer is truly better, for which patients, and under what circumstances.

At this point, it is not altogether clear which elements of extended treatments are the most important. As was discussed in chapter 2, many individuals with substance use disorders have psychological, biological, and social or environmental challenges that leave them at heightened vulnerability to relapse for extended periods of time. The key therapeutic elements common to most forms of effective continuing care—structure, social support, monitoring, skill building and problem solving, empowerment, connections to other sources of support in the community, and linkage to services for co-occurring problems—help patients better manage the vulnerabilities that they will never entirely leave behind, even when in recovery for long periods. Longer continuing care may work simply because it extends the duration of this assistance.

Active Efforts to Reach and Retain Patients Are Crucial

As was observed in chapter 3, one of the notable similarities between the successful extended interventions reviewed in that chapter was that none of them relied on patients to simply show up at a treatment clinic week after week. Rather, each approach involved taking the intervention to the patient, by involving a spouse or partner, visiting the home, using the telephone to deliver the intervention, aggressively finding patients and getting them back into treatment when necessary, or actively handing off patients from one level of care to the next. This observation certainly held true with regard to other successful continuing care models reviewed in subsequent chapters.

Thus, we have an interesting paradox regarding the goals of continuing care and the methods necessary to get there. Ultimately, continuing care strives to equip each patient to manage his or her own recovery by engaging in regular self-monitoring, using active coping methods, and establishing and maintaining strong connections to support systems in the community (Institute of Medicine [IOM], 2006; Wagner et al., 2001). However, getting to that point requires active efforts on the part of clinicians to deliver the ingredients of continuing care that will ultimately help bring about these new self-directed behaviors in the patient. It is the rare individual who will faithfully come to the treatment clinic every week to receive extended care. As was reported earlier, only 36% of admissions complete IOP or OP, and median lengths of stay are under 90 days (Substance Abuse and Mental Health Services Administration, 2008). It is quite clear that keeping patients engaged in continuing care over longer periods of time requires outreach efforts of one sort or another, as well as interventions that place a lower burden on that person and his or her family.

Incentives Are Effective

Research reviewed in this book indicates that retention in extended continuing care can also be improved by providing concrete incentives to patients for attendance at sessions. Although higher value incentives probably work best, there is ample evidence that relatively low-cost incentives provided to patients or counselors can have a significant effect (Chutuape, Katz, & Stitzer, 2001; Lash et al., 2007; Shepard et al., 2006). These findings are consistent with recent meta-analyses of the research literature on the effectiveness of contingency management and other interventions that provide incentives for abstinence or attendance (Lussier, Heil, Mongeon, Badger, & Higgins, 2006; Prendergast, Podus, Finney, Greenwell, & Roll, 2006).

Reactions to the well-documented efficacy of contingency management and other incentive-based interventions have been mixed, with some counselors and policymakers—not to mention some in the general public—objecting to the idea of paying patients with substance use disorders "to do what they should be doing anyway." This is another argument for pursuing further work on lower cost incentives, such as the social recognition approach used by Lash et al. (2007). Moreover, focusing the incentives on counselor performance or the performance of an entire clinic, rather than on that of the patients, may also be less controversial (McLellan, Kemp, Brooks, & Carise, 2008). However, economic analyses may ultimately show that paying patients for abstinence or attendance in continuing care through contingency management is the most cost-effective method for improving outcomes.

Linkage to Other Supports Improves Outcomes

Most continuing care interventions are directed primarily toward changing the patient's cognitions, emotions, and behaviors. However, this focus on the patient may be of limited benefit over the long haul. People in recovery also need a community of support—family members, friends, employers, and peers from mutual help organizations who will provide a safe and nurturing environment for recovery (White, 2008, 2009; White & Kurtz, 2006). The work of Litt, Kadden, Kabela-Cormier, and Petry (2007) and Timko, DeBenedetti, and Billow (2006) demonstrates treatment interventions can help patients to develop new social networks that are more supportive of abstinence and to become more engaged in those social supports. The recovery coach approaches described in chapter 12 also pay particular attention to developing a strong social support network for recovery and setting up open lines of communication so that social support is readily available should the patient show signs of increased vulnerability to relapse.

Theoretical Orientation and Intensity May Not Be Important

Another conclusion from the research reviewed in this book is that the theoretical orientation of the therapy or counseling may not matter as much as how it is provided. Most effective continuing care interventions strive in one way or another to increase coping skills, but there appears to be at least several ways to accomplish this. Given the high dropout rate, the degree to which an intervention fosters sustained involvement is probably much more important than how it goes about trying to create and sustain behavior change. Similarly, intensity of continuing care also did not seem terribly important, at least for typical patients. However, some research suggests that patients who are doing poorly in the first phase of treatment will do better with more intensive continuing care (McKay, Lynch, Shepard, & Pettinati, 2005).

CHALLENGES TO IMPROVING CONTINUING CARE

The research reviewed here also highlights some of the challenges that need to be addressed to improve the acceptability and effectiveness of continuing care interventions. These challenges include the need to focus to a greater degree in continuing care development efforts on providing something of greater value to patients, making more progress on adaptive models of care, arriving at a better understanding of the processes of change, developing fiscal mechanisms to support extended care models, and developing integrated models of care that involve primary care and other service delivery systems.

Moving Beyond Deprivation Approaches to Continuing Care

Most interventions in the addictions are derived from what could be labeled a *deprivation* model of treatment. That is, these treatments are designed to help those with substance use disorders live without their substances of abuse, or at least with considerably reduced levels of use. For example, cognitive–behavioral therapy (CBT) is focused on teaching people skills to cope with various stressors without using alcohol or drugs, self-help programs such as Alcoholics Anonymous (AA) provide spiritual and social supports for living an abstinent life, and the group-based interventions that are offered in the vast majority of addiction treatment programs use education as well as peer pressure and support to advocate for the benefits of living without alcohol and drugs. Moreover, the medications that are available to treat alcoholism are designed to make the alcoholic sick if he or she drinks (i.e., disulfiram) or to reduce the pleasure of drinking (i.e., naltrexone). Granted, the behavioral interventions also try to provide something positive to the individual with a substance use disorder—namely, the benefits associated with an abstinent lifestyle. However, the emphasis is clearly on taking away something that has been of considerable importance to the patient.

This model appears to work quite well when people are in a crisis and the costs associated with continued alcohol or drug use are overwhelmingly high. It also works well for people who, for whatever combination of reasons, are truly ready to commit to an abstinent lifestyle. However, many of those with substance use disorders are not interested in this sort of approach and therefore never enter treatment. An even more relevant concern, given the focus of this book, is that acceptance of and enthusiasm for a deprivation-based approach is likely to wane after a few months of treatment, when the negative consequences of the crisis that drove the person into treatment have subsided somewhat. At times, the ability of individuals with substance use disorders to forget "how bad it really was" is truly remarkable.

The fact that most of the available treatments for addiction focus on taking away something of value to individuals with substance use disorders suggests that a key goal of our efforts to develop better continuing care should be to make ongoing participation in treatment considerably more appealing. Several approaches to addiction treatment have attempted to do just that. As discussed previously, contingency management interventions provide incentives that are tied to good performance in treatment, specifically drug-free urine tests or attendance (Higgins et al., 2003; Lussier et al., 2006; Petry, Alessi, & Hanson, 2007; Prendergast et al., 2006). The incentives are usually gift certificates that can be used to obtain goods and services that are consistent with recovery. The community reinforcement approach tries to make abstinence more appealing than continued use by providing incentives for good performance, services to improve key relationships, help with employment, and access to substance-free social clubs (Meyers & Smith, 1995). Couples therapy strives to alter interactions between an alcohol or drug addict and his or her romantic partner so that the partner engages in a pleasing manner with the addict when he or she is abstinent and withdraws when substance use occurs (O'Farrell & Fals-Stewart, 2001). Some research programs, described earlier in this book, have provided employment or housing, contingent on abstinence from alcohol and drugs (Milby et al., 2000, 2003; Silverman et al., 2002).

AA promises those who join the organization that the act of giving up alcohol and other drugs will lead to a greatly enriched and happier life. Some participants clearly find this to be the case. For these individuals, involvement in AA becomes an entrée to an entirely new life, complete with devoted friends, the experience of belonging and acceptance, the opportunity to help others, a renewed sense of purpose and meaning, and even romantic possibilities and employment opportunities. In these cases, being deprived of alcohol or drugs can seem like a relatively small price to pay. However, most individuals who try AA do not experience these benefits, often because they stop attending before the benefits can be realized.

It is highly illuminating to contrast the relative efficacy, effectiveness, and popularity of two pharmacological approaches to opiate addiction, naltrexone and methadone. Naltrexone has the potential to be 100% efficacious in the treatment of opiate addiction because it completely blocks opiate receptors. A person who takes naltrexone every day cannot get high on opiates, no matter how much of the drug is consumed. However, naltrexone has been a miserable failure in the treatment of opiate dependence because addicts simply do not want to take it. The medication completely eliminates the pleasurable aspects of opiate use but provides nothing in return. Methadone, in contrast, is not 100% effective in blocking the positive effects of opiate use. However, because it is an opiate receptor agonist rather than an antagonist, it provides a milder opiate-like effect, which addicts tend to like. Therefore, it has been a popular treatment for opiate dependence, and there are often waiting lists at clinics that provide it. One of the great ironies in addiction treatment is that we already have efficacious medications that nearly eliminate the use of alcohol and opiates—the only problem is that few people want to take them for very long.

All of this suggests that we need to move past deprivation models of care to devise ways to provide incentives of one sort or another to those in recovery. This will no doubt require considerable effort and will need to go beyond simple contingency management interventions that provide goods and services when patients provide drug-free urines. The work of Milby and Silverman and their colleagues (Milby et al., 2000, 2003; Silverman et al., 2002, 2004) suggests that even the most severe addicts can become abstinent when opportunities for housing and employment are provided. Families and communities may need to join together in efforts to identify and supply desirable incentives that can be provided when patients stick with continuing care and achieve sustained abstinence. Creative, "out of the box" thinking is needed in this process. It is likely that some amount of tailoring will be necessary to provide the kind of incentives that will be most powerful for a particular person. For example, adaptive protocols could be designed in which failure to respond to one type of incentive would lead to a switch to another family of possible incentives.

Finally, we may be able to make treatment more appealing by increasing the focus on the identification, facilitation, and strengthening of patients' existing skills, interests, and talents (McKay, 2001b). Although these issues are clearly important in promoting extended recovery, more rapid attention to them might be beneficial, at least with some individuals. Consider a person whose whole world has come to revolve around cocaine use. A standard treatment approach would focus on trying to create some distance between the individual and that world, by urging him to spend as much time as possible in treatment settings, get immersed in self-help, and live in a halfway house with others in recovery. However, a crash course in finding other activities that are engrossing, fun, and otherwise rewarding may help make the prospect of another day without cocaine more palatable. Writing on how health behavior changes are maintained, Rothman (2000) observed that fear of negative consequences may help someone stop smoking or using alcohol and drugs, but enjoyment of the benefits that these behavior changes might bring are probably necessary to sustain changes in health behaviors.

Improving Adaptive Algorithms

Much of this book has been devoted to describing adaptive continuing care interventions, reviewing their effectiveness, outlining how they are developed and evaluated, and noting their limitations. Arguably, the most important issues in improving adaptive continuing care algorithms are figuring out how to retain patients when they are not doing well and assembling treatment alternatives that are different enough that patients who have a poor response to one intervention may still respond to a second or third choice from the available menu.

With regard to the former, it is possible that providing patients with a range of treatment choices and incentives might help to retain them in continuing care if they begin to use again or otherwise lose motivation for further treatment. With patients who have more intact social connections and better employment histories, the benefits of retaining a professional career can be a powerful incentive to comply with changes in treatment when the original plan is not working. As was described in chapter 5, this is certainly the case with physicians and pilots. However, the work of Brooner and Kidorf (2002) clearly demonstrates that people without such high-level employment opportunities will also comply with adaptive modifications to treatment when continued access to something that they want is dependent on it.

In many ways, the tasks of developing a range of effective treatment options and providing something of value to patients so that they are more willing to hang in there when the going gets tough are closely related. Patients may not want to pick between cognitive–behavioral therapy, 12-step facilitation, or motivational interviewing, or even between a behavioral intervention and a medication. Rather, they may want to focus on something entirely different from their addiction, such as housing, financial matters, employment, hobbies or recreational activities, skills and talents, parenting or child-care issues, or family functioning. Patients may also want a goal of sharply reduced use, rather than abstinence, or prefer regular monitoring of biological signs of use rather than counseling in a clinic setting. Further work is needed to develop algorithms that will provide more appealing augmentations or switches to standard addiction treatment when patient motivation for treatment or abstinence (or both) begins to wane. However, one of the challenges here is to not engineer in perverse incentives that reward poor progress (e.g., patients become eligible for incentives for participation if they relapse or fail to attend sessions). Another exciting area of investigation in adaptive treatment is the development of methods to apply newer assessment technology (Gustafson et al., 2005; Shiffman & Waters, 2004) to promote more frequent assessment of tailoring variables and consequently more rapid modifications of treatment when necessary.

In any case, we are clearly moving past the old model, in which continuing care was reserved only for those who successfully completed their first phase of care. One could envision an adaptive system in which prior treatment response (e.g., cost of addiction treatment in the prior year) and response to the current episode (e.g., early dropout, completion but with poor overall progress, completion with good progress) would be used to determine the approach to continuing care provided. Patients who completed their first phase of care with good progress would go into telephone contact or a combination of face-to-face counseling and telephone contacts. Conversely, high-cost patients would go into more intensive case management interventions similar to those evaluated by Morgenstern et al. (2006). Early dropouts would be offered a choice of models in the hope of promoting engagement in some form of treatment.

The other cutting-edge challenge in adaptive treatment concerns the development of methods and study designs that will support sequential randomization without requiring sample sizes that are simply beyond what is currently affordable. Work in these areas is proceeding and will no doubt eventually yield better study designs and more exact estimates of needed sample sizes (L. M. Collins et al., 2007; L. M. Collins, Murphy, Nair, & Strecher, 2005).

Determining How People Change and Maintain Change While in Continuing Care

There has been surprisingly little research on processes of change in continuing care. Although more studies are needed that test hypotheses about specific mediators (e.g., Mensinger, Lynch, Ten Have, & McKay, 2007), we likely need to go back to the drawing board to study what actually happens in treatment sessions between clinicians and patients (Kazdin & Nock, 2003; McKay, 2006; Morgenstern & McKay, 2007; Moyers, Miller, & Hendrickson, 2005). The work of Karno and Longabaugh (2003, 2004, 2005a, 2005b) on interactions between patient characteristics and counselor style in Project MATCH (Matching Alcohol Treatments to Client Heterogeneity) is an excellent example of how this sort of work can pay off. There is also a pressing need for study of the role of Patient × Therapist interactions in patient compliance with stepped care and other recommended changes in adaptive protocols.

Understanding the Preferences and Choices of Patients

We think that providing a wider range of services, extending the duration of the interventions, making the treatments more user friendly and accessible, and so forth will make our continuing care models more appealing and effective. However, we know little about how patients perceive our efforts to improve continuing care or what they actually want in this regard. We simply have not asked them. This is due to several factors, including the widespread belief that information from such "customer satisfaction" surveys was of little value and the generally lower regard most treatment researchers have had for qualitative data. Another major limitation was that the people whom we most needed to talk with, those who dropped out of treatment, were difficult to find and interview.

Fortunately, there is now much more interest in patient preferences and perspectives and better methods for gathering and evaluating such data. Moreover, social scientists such as Phillipe Bourgois have pioneered efforts to gather standardized information systematically from out-of-treatment populations (Bourgois et al., 2006). These new methods make it possible to study issues such as why patients stop attending continuing care, what they might find helpful if they start to use alcohol or drugs again, what might get them back involved with treatment of some sort, and so forth. Future research on new continuing care models should involve interdisciplinary teams that include anthropologists or other social scientists who can gather critical information on patient preference and reactions to the interventions.

Financial Issues—"Paying for It"

A recent article by Popovici, French, and McKay (2008) reviewed studies that have examined the cost-effectiveness or cost-benefit of continuing care interventions. This review identified 11 such studies, most of which focused on postrelease continuing care interventions for individuals with substance use disorders who received an initial phase of treatment while incarcerated. The authors concluded that the findings from this relatively small number of studies, each with certain data or methodological limitations, suggest that continuing care models that encompass different modalities of treatment can be more effective from an economic standpoint than acute care models, in which patients are treated with a single intervention approach. Adding elements of continuing care to various addiction treatment programs seems to enhance their effectiveness, thereby yielding positive net economic benefits. Although good research in this area is hard to come by, simulation studies may be able to accomplish what usually requires an expensive and lengthy data collection process (Zarkin, Dunlap, Hicks, & Mamo, 2005).

Continuing care is a popular concept in addiction treatment, and there is some evidence of cost-effectiveness and cost-benefit for it, as shown by studies reviewed in the Popovici et al. (2008) article. However, one of the major challenges to any attempts to improve and extend continuing care models is finding mechanisms to pay for the additional services. This is all the more the case following the economic crisis of 2008–2009. In discussions with state directors of addiction services, it is clear that there will likely be no new funds forthcoming for addiction treatment, and therefore increasing continuing care services will require cost shifting. This might be possible, if providing additional extended continuing care leads to better overall addiction disease management and less use of high-cost acute care services. Moreover, there is great interest in showing through research that good continuing care and addiction disease management lead to reductions in costs for other state agencies, such as welfare and criminal justice. Documentation of such savings provides a strong rationale for shifting some of the funding from these agencies into addiction treatment. This has been already done successfully in Washington state.

There is also evidence of a growing belief on the part of policymakers and those agencies that fund addiction treatment that continuing care is a good investment. For example, new billing codes are available in some states that make it possible to receive payment for telephone sessions and other types of extended monitoring. Directors of addiction services at the local and state levels can also decide to create payment structures that provide incentives to programs for successfully engaging and retaining patients in continuing care. For example, Delaware recently enacted a pilot program in which detoxification programs could earn a bonus if they reached targets related to percentage of patients who were successfully transitioned to treatment after leaving short-term detoxification programs. Finally, new mental health parity legislation may ultimately provide better insurance coverage for extended care in the addictions, although this is certainly not the case at present.

Integration of Continuing Care With Current Treatment Approaches

Two of the more important unresolved questions with new continuing care models are where they should be located and how they should be staffed

(Miller & Weisner, 2002). One solution is to locate continuing care providers within specialty programs and have the regular program counselors deliver the interventions. This, in fact, is how most continuing care is provided at this time. However, this approach breaks down to some degree when continuing care is extended over longer periods of time. Counselors may not have enough time to provide both intensive interventions such as IOP and extended continuing care to the same patients without fairly drastic changes in program staffing patterns. What happens when a patient needs more intensive treatment at a subsequent point, but does not want to go back to the original treatment program? Does the original counselor stay involved in some way with treatment? Moreover, for how long is the original program ethically and legally responsible for the patient during extended continuing care?

Another possible solution, at least in urban and suburban areas, would be to establish recovery centers with their own staff that would accept patients from multiple initial treatment programs in the area and provide extended continuing care and recovery support services. Such recovery centers have been established in a number of locations, including the state of Connecticut and the city of Philadelphia, and they make use of both professionals and peers to deliver job-skills training, telephone monitoring and support, help with housing, and other recovery support services.

Collaborating With Other Treatment Systems to Provide Continuing Care

There is also considerable interest in developing and implementing service delivery models in which continuing care for substance use disorders is integrated with medically oriented treatment in primary care clinics and other medical practices (Miller & Weisner, 2002). There are several major advantages to this approach. Such clinics already provide ongoing management of medical disorders, often over periods of many years. Therefore, they are well suited to coordinating care for chronic disorders and arranging for adaptive changes in treatment when the current approach is no longer working. In addition, medical clinics are in a much better position to prescribe and monitor medications for addiction and co-occurring medical and psychiatric problems. It is known from research by Willenbring and Olson (1999), Weisner et al. (2001), and others that integrated care models are more effective in delivering medical services to patients with substance use disorders than traditional models of care and foster higher rates of sustained compliance. One of the challenges that will have to be addressed concerns who has ultimate clinical responsibility and liability for patients as they progress through various components of continuing care, which might be provided within different agencies or even across different systems (e.g., addiction specialty care, medical primary care).

Finally, there is a good chance that a greater number of effective medications for addiction will be developed in the coming years, and vaccines for cocaine and other drugs are also possible (Martell, Mitchell, Poling, Gonsai, & Kosten, 2005; Sofuoglu & Kosten, 2006). There is likely, therefore, to be an increasing need for continuing care protocols that combine effective behavioral and pharmacological interventions as new medications come on line. Kathleen Carroll and colleagues at Yale have done pioneering work in the development and evaluation of these combination interventions (Carroll et al., 2004; Carroll, Nich, Ball, McCance, & Rounsaville, 1998). The medical management intervention tested in the COMBINE study (Pettinati et al., 2004) is another example of a treatment protocol that combines behavioral and pharmacological interventions. Further work is needed to extend these models into the continuing care phase of treatment and to develop adaptive protocols that make use of both behavioral and pharmacological treatments. Given the lack of physicians and nurses in traditional addiction specialty care programs, it is likely that integrated programs based in medical settings may be much better service delivery sites for these initiatives.

VISION FOR OPTIMAL CONTINUING CARE

A conference at the Betty Ford Institute in the fall of 2007 that focused on continuing care brought together clinicians, treatment researchers, treatment program directors, state agency directors, representatives of industry employee assistance programs and physicians' health plans, recovery coaches, and people in recovery and their family members. The goal of the conference was to produce position statements on the key components of effective continuing care and on the issues and problems that still need to be addressed in the field. The following components were identified as essential for good continuing care (McKay, Carise, et al., 2009):

- regular objective monitoring of alcohol and drug use status that goes beyond patient self-report;
- a community or circle of recovery for the patient, consisting of important stakeholders in that person's recovery;
- active case management or coaching to monitor progress, coordinate the circle of recovery, and arrange for additional treatment for co-occurring problems as needed;
- transparency and open communication among the patient, coaches and treatment providers, and other members of the circle of recovery with regard to the patient's progress or lack thereof; and
- involvement in AA or other mutual-help organizations.

These conclusions were influenced to some degree by the success of intensive programs for physicians and pilots, which all involve close supervision of the patient, extended monitoring of substance use with urine toxicology screens, and transparency between stakeholders with regard to the patient's progress.

The common goal of these programs is to construct an environment in which the person in recovery essentially has "nowhere to hide." These programs are clearly offered with compassion and are dedicated to bringing about recovery. However, they see the person with a substance use disorder as his own worst enemy—someone who must be protected from his tendencies to sneak off and use alcohol or drugs whenever close supervision is lifted or to provide false or inconsistent reports to those who care about him and his recovery. Although patients with substance use disorders certainly engage in these kinds of behaviors, one has to wonder about how much an intervention of this sort is likely to appeal to prospective patients—especially if they are not threatened with the potential loss of a high-paying job such as being a physician or pilot. For example, how many people would voluntarily agree to regular urine testing if there were no severe consequences—such as loss of a license to practice medicine or a return to prison—for refusing to be involved with the program? For an extended continuing care model to yield positive results, it has to be efficacious, and people have to be willing to participate in it. Our experience with naltrexone for opiate addicts and disulfiram for alcoholics all too clearly illustrates that point.

By comparison, several other approaches to continuing care place a much greater priority on patient self-determination. These include the recovery movement and motivational interviewing, as well as some aspects of Wagner et al.'s (2001) chronic care model and IOM (2001, 2006) recommendations regarding needed changes to the health system. These approaches stress the need to involve patients more actively in their treatments by making participation more appealing and providing a greater range of choices.

The adaptive approach to continuing care described in this book has elements of both of these treatment models. Like programs for physicians and pilots, adaptive treatment requires the frequent—and valid—assessment of tailoring variables to keep close track of patient progress. However, this approach recognizes that patients are unlikely to continue to attend such programs unless they are clearly getting something positive by participating or at least avoiding something highly undesirable. In reality, most patients are not faced with the latter, or at least will not be over extended periods of time. Therefore, the adaptive approach instead focuses on trying to make treatment more attractive by incorporating patient choice and preference, reducing the burden of treatment when possible, and providing therapeutic options when the current treatment approach is not working well.

This book has traced the evolution of continuing care for substance use disorders from the "one size fits all" group counseling model that has dominated the field for many years to newer approaches that combine greater flexibility, the use of other modalities and forms of service delivery, a wider range of strategies and techniques to foster higher rates of engagement and retention, and extended durations of care. These new models are also much more focused on regular assessment of patient status and progress and the use of those data to adjust, or adapt, treatment over time. Further developments in the accuracy, efficiency, and portability of monitoring tools and devices will no doubt increase the flexibility and effectiveness of adaptive continuing care protocols. Moreover, advances in pharmacotherapies for alcohol and drug use disorders will further improve these protocols, particularly if a wider range of effective medications with different mechanisms of action becomes available.

As has been outlined here, there are still a number of difficult challenges to overcome in the development of adaptive continuing care protocols. These challenges include problems with retention, availability of enough effective treatment alternatives, and questions regarding how best to staff and fund these interventions. However, there is still good reason for considerable optimism regarding the future of disease management in the addictions on the basis of the results of the innovative continuing care and disease management studies that have been described here.

As a closing note, advances in monitoring technology, computerized service delivery modalities, and medications should not obscure the fact that continuing care at its core still primarily involves a relationship between a patient and a caregiver. Although incentives and more flexible, lower burden interventions may increase rates of participation, the clinician's personal qualities, therapeutic skills, and ability to form a strong working alliance with the patient also have an important influence on whether the patient elects to stay involved with continuing care or drop out. Therefore, as work to improve continuing care moves forward on the service delivery system, information technology, and pharmacological fronts, it will be crucial not to overlook the need also to concentrate on improving the ability of clinicians to form and sustain strong therapeutic connections with patients.

APPENDIX: PROVIDING TELEPHONE-BASED ADAPTIVE CONTINUING CARE

This appendix presents material from the telephone continuing care protocols that we have been using in studies at the University of Pennsylvania, as described in this book. The material includes a guide to the face-to-face orientation session with patients at the beginning of the protocol, a detailed description of the material to be covered in each telephone contact, the brief assessment that is used to monitor risk and protective factors at the start of each session, and a description of how to conduct a face-to-face evaluation session when stepped care appears necessary. These materials were developed in collaboration with Deborah Van Horn and Rebecca Morrison. A more complete version of this protocol, along with other support materials, is forthcoming from Hazelden Press.

If possible, it is recommended that patients begin this protocol before graduating from their initial treatment program to increase the likelihood that they will make a successful transition to continuing care. Given the high rate of dropout in most outpatient programs, it is important to engage the patient in the telephone protocol before he or she either graduates or drops out of the initial phase of care. During the period of overlap, when the patient is still attending an intensive outpatient program (IOP) or outpatient program (OP) and having telephone sessions, the calls place a greater emphasis on supporting continued engagement in that program. This is done by addressing (a) barriers to attendance, such as problems with transportation, family roles, or employment; (b) diminishing motivation for treatment or recovery; or (c) problems with the IOP or OP itself.

GENERAL COMMENTS ON TELEPHONE CONTINUING CARE

Before proceeding with specific information about the protocol, some general remarks are in order. Telephone-based continuing care (TEL) is less burdensome to patients, and most patients report that they like this form of treatment delivery. However, it can also be more difficult for therapists to deliver because of the lack of access to nonverbal cues. There is also less of a margin for error, given that the sessions are short and it is more difficult to reconnect with a patient over the telephone if a rupture to the therapeutic alliance occurs. Attention to the following factors will facilitate the successful delivery of telephone continuing care.

Creating and Maintaining a Therapeutic Alliance on the Telephone

As much as possible, phone call appointments should be at the same time each week, and the counselor's consistency and availability at that time set an important tone and also serve to communicate to the patient the importance of the phone sessions. Counselors must also be careful to note any signs of trouble in what is either said or not said by the patient and should address these issues rather than ignore them.

It is important to give patients plenty of positive comments about what they are doing with regard to their treatment, including calling on time, having their patient workbook with them, filling out the progress assessment form before the session, and so forth. Counselors should listen for changes in behavior patterns that might indicate cause for concern, particularly behaviors or experiences the patient has identified as red flags (discussed in the Orientation to Telephone Continuing Care section). Initially, the phone sessions may feel awkward because of the newness, brevity, and the structure of the protocol. To keep the telephone sessions sounding fresh and spontaneous, as opposed to overly scripted, it is best if counselors develop their own approach to covering the required material. What we provide here are sample scripts that might be useful in developing such an approach.

Finally, some counselors are initially uncomfortable working with a patient whom they cannot directly observe or from whom they cannot obtain urine samples to verify reports of abstinence. Our experience is that patients will admit to problems, including substance use, during telephone calls, although underreporting certainly happens. In these cases, patients invariably end up conveying that they are in trouble, usually by missing scheduled telephone calls or sounding superficial or avoidant on calls they do make. An experienced addiction counselor will quickly figure out what is happening. As is described later, we often invite patients in for face-to-face sessions—and ask for a urine sample—if we have reason to believe that they have started using alcohol or drugs again. The important point is that the maintenance of an alliance in a TEL intervention requires that the counselor act on concerns and not succumb to the temptation to let something go without addressing it.

Establishing a Recovery Support Structure

In addition to consistency of telephone appointments, other necessary structures to be established early in treatment include the patient's regular attendance at Alcoholics Anonymous (AA), Narcotics Anonymous, or other types of support groups and his or her ability to talk with another sober person before, during, or after the meetings, as well as some other established way for the patient to experience meaningful social contact, such as participation at church, work, family contact, school or a training program, involvement with a pet, and so forth. The counselor's awareness of the establishment and use of these structures will make it easier to listen for the development of any cracks in the structure(s), which should be interpreted as potential red flags.

Assessing Risk and Protective Factors

Each telephone contact should start with a structured assessment of current risks and protective factors. In one of our current cocaine continuing care studies, for example, we assess three general factors (i.e., recent alcohol or drug use, HIV risk behavior, and attendance at any current face-to-face treatment); five risk factors (i.e., compliance with medical or psychiatric treatment, depression, self-efficacy, craving, and being in high-risk situations); and five protective factors (i.e., coping efforts in high-risk situations, sober social or leisure activities, pursuit of personal goals, self-help meetings, and contact with a sponsor). Data gathered in this brief progress assessment are used to monitor current status, note changes in symptoms and functioning, select issues to focus on in the rest of the session, guide decisions about possible changes in level of care, and trigger case management efforts. This assessment brings considerable structure to the telephone sessions and helps to keep them from turning into chat sessions.

Using Cognitive–Behavioral Therapy Techniques

Our telephone protocol makes use of a number of techniques from cognitive–behavioral therapy. These include the identification of risky situations, learning to anticipate such situations, developing better coping responses for these situations, and rehearsing those coping responses during the call. From our experience, this is often more difficult to do over the telephone than in person. Thus, the counselor may have to keep pointing out when the patient is being vague and omitting important details about risky situations and coping attempts while on the telephone.

ORIENTATION TO TELEPHONE CONTINUING CARE

Before beginning telephone continuing care, the counselor should have one or two 45-minute face-to-face sessions with the patient to explain how the telephone protocol works. This is also a time for the patient to raise questions. However, the most important task in these sessions is for the counselor and patient to establish enough of a connection and rapport that the patient will feel comfortable talking about potentially painful material on the calls and will feel that the counselor can be a helpful ally in the recovery process.

During the session, the counselor should

- acknowledge the patient's progress so far in treatment and discuss any concerns;
- explain the telephone-based treatment, with a strong emphasis on the importance of completing each phone call, doing self-

monitoring between calls and any homework that is suggested, and being willing to report substance use if it occurs and ask for help when necessary; and

- explain the adaptive protocol that allows for modifications to treatment over time on the basis of how the patient is doing.

The counselor next guides the patient in choosing high-risk situations and recovery activities (i.e., protective factors) to monitor and in selecting relevant between-session goals. The counselor should stress the importance of being as proactive as possible in managing addiction by engaging in more recovery-oriented behaviors and activities and being alert to the emergence of relapse triggers and other problems in early stages before they lead to relapse. The counselor should also

- complete a crisis plan with the patient that outlines a series of steps the patient can take when a crisis or emergency occurs,
- review the Progress Assessment Worksheet with the patient during the session,
- clarify anything the patient does not understand about the telephone protocol and the progress assessment worksheet and discuss any misgivings he or she may have about following through with the protocol,
- provide feedback based on the patient's responses on the progress assessment worksheet,
- ask the patient what high-risk situations he or she anticipates facing in the interval before the first phone session and briefly address possible coping behaviors for those situations,
- identify one goal for the patient to work on before the first phone session, and
- schedule the first phone session within the next week.

One important question is, Who should be responsible for initiating the calls—the patient or the counselor? There are pros and cons for each option. Asking the patient to initiate the call communicates the counselor's confidence in the patient's capacity to follow through with his or her commitment to the protocol and improve his or her life situation. It also sends a clear message that the patient is responsible for her own recovery. Moreover, it allows the patient to call in from wherever she happens to be at the scheduled time, rather than having to be at a designated place at the time of the call. Therefore, holding the patient accountable for her role in the telephone contact should not be viewed as punitive, demeaning, or an infringement on her autonomy. However, busy counselors may have difficulty accommodating late calls. In our experience, patients do not call when they are scheduled to at least 50% of the time, and in those cases the counselor has to call in an attempt to locate the patient and complete the scheduled session.

Therefore, we develop a call completion plan with the patient during the orientation session. This process involves exploring the patient's access to telephones, preference around calling in or being called, contingency plans for times when initial attempts to complete a call fail, and so forth. The patient is advised that she and her counselor will revisit this issue frequently during the protocol, in case modifications are necessary. The goal is to do whatever it takes to increase the likelihood of completed calls.

The counselor should also explain to the patient why increases in level of care may be recommended at some point and how the telephone sessions will be used to make that decision. The counselor should stress that a recommendation for increased level of care is not a punishment. Rather, the counselor and the patient are working together to improve the patient's substance abuse status, and if the current approach to treatment is not working as well as it should, another approach needs to be tried. The counselor might say something such as this:

> If you went to your doctor because of an infection and the first medication she gave you didn't seem to be doing the job, you would want your doctor to increase the amount of the medication, add another medication to the one you were taking, or switch medications entirely. You would expect the doctor to keep adjusting your treatment until you got better.

Obviously, treatment for substance abuse is different from that for infections in many ways, not the least of which is that stepped-up treatment usually requires a lot more work than switching medications. However, the counselor may be able to increase the willingness of the patient to go along with changes in the treatment protocol if an emphasis is placed on the message that "we're in this together, and let's see if making these changes will help you achieve your goals more quickly."

DETAILED INSTRUCTIONS AND SAMPLE SCRIPTS
FOR TELEPHONE SESSIONS

Our protocol for telephone continuing care sessions has nine steps, which are presented in Exhibit A.1 and outlined in this section. In our experience, it takes between 15 and 30 minutes to complete the protocol, depending on whether there have been any recent crises and what else comes up in the progress assessment, as well has how talkative the patient is.

1. Acknowledge the patient for completing the call, and orient to the task at hand.

Because the telephone sessions are brief, the counselor should quickly check to see whether there have been any emergencies since the last contact

EXHIBIT A.1
Outline of Telephone Counseling Sessions

1. Acknowledge patient for the call, and orient to the task at hand.
2. Review progress assessment items.
3. Provide feedback on risk level; suggest change in level of care if warranted.
4. Review progress and goals from last call.
5. Identify upcoming high-risk situations.
6. Select target for remainder of call.
7. Conduct brief problem solving regarding target concern(s).
8. Set goal(s) for interval before next call.
9. Schedule next phone call.

and, if not, move into the progress assessment. However, some more casual conversation is fine, as long as it is kept short. Here is an example of how the call might begin:

> Thanks for calling in on time. Are there any emergencies I should know about? OK, let's get right into your progress assessment worksheet. Do you have that material with you now? Did you complete it before the call?

- If the patient did not call in on time or has missed one or more scheduled calls, reinforce the patient for resuming calls and mention that you will address scheduling issues later.
- If there is an emergency, ask the patient to describe it briefly. In most cases, it will be enough to assure him that it will be discussed further after completing the progress assessment. If the patient is upset, it may be necessary to deal with the emergency situation before returning to the structure of the call.

2. Review progress assessment items.

The current version of our progress assessment consists of three items on current status (i.e., recent alcohol or drug use, HIV risk behavior, and attendance at any current face-to-face treatment), five risk factor items, and five protective factor items. Sample items from this assessment are presented in Table A.1.

- Complete the progress assessment items in order, beginning with "Did you use any alcohol or drugs over the past week?"
- Record the patient's responses. Be alert to how the patient's responses bear on his stated goals since the last session and to longer term treatment goals. Is he showing progress over time toward a prorecovery lifestyle?
- Continually reinforce the patient for sticking with the process and providing complete and accurate information, even when it is not all good news.

Thanks for being so honest with me. That's the only way we can tell where you are doing well and where you might need to change.

Our newest version of the progress assessment provides guidance to therapists and counselors on adaptive modifications to session content and case management efforts linked to each item in the assessment. For example, adaptive treatment for patients who report depression involves providing relapse prevention (RP) focused specifically on coping with depressed mood as a potential relapse trigger and CBT-informed advice for mild depression. Case management for depressed mood involves referral and linkage to mental health treatment, if the patient is not already receiving such care.

3. Provide feedback on risk level.

On the basis of the scoring of the progress assessment form, the counselor should give the patient feedback on relapse risk level. Typically, patients with low scores on the risk items and high scores on the protective items are at low risk, those with moderate scores on risk items and low to moderate scores on protective items are at moderate risk, and those with high scores on risk items coupled with low scores on protective items are at high risk. However, it is important to consider how the patient has looked over the past several contacts and to note worrisome patterns, such as an increase over several weeks in risk factors and a concurrent decline in protective factors. A more detailed discussion of various approaches to scoring risk is included at the end of this appendix. The counselor should place the feedback in the context of the patient's goals since the last session and overall treatment goals and include suggestions for change in level of care if warranted.

Low Risk

Given what you've told me, you are doing a great job of keeping yourself at low risk of relapse. You have not been using and have not had strong urges to use, your degree of confidence in being able to manage stress remains high, and you're still talking with your sponsor and spending almost no time in risky situations.

Moderate Risk

You've been spending more time around people who are using and getting to fewer AA meetings. You've told me that combination has gotten you in trouble before. I am concerned that you are now at a moderate risk for relapse, and one thing we can discuss in our time today is how stepping up our phone calls can help you get back on track.

High Risk

Given what you've told me, you are having more cravings and are very concerned about staying away from alcohol and drugs. That gets me concerned, too, that you may be at high risk for relapse. Let's think about

TABLE A.1

Examples of Items From the Progress Assessment for Adaptive Telephone Continuing Care

Item	Scoring	Patient's score (circle)	Adaptive modifications	Case management guidelines
General status items: Each contributes to adaptive care decisions, but scores are not added up.				
Since we last spoke on ____, how many days have you been clean from cocaine? From alcohol? From other drugs?	*No substance use* = 0 *Any substance use* = 1	0 1	*Slip:* Debrief and support successful RP efforts, increase frequency of contact *Relapse:* Debrief, focus on reattainment of abstinence, increase frequency of contact, in-person sessions	Encourage patient to discuss relapse in IOP. Encourage patient to return to/reengage in IOP, if applicable. Encourage patient to enter inpatient treatment or detox if needed.
Risk factors: high score = more risk				
How often have you felt depressed or like you had no interest in anything? How long did it last? *Probe for sustained depression.*	*No depression* = 0 *Depressed less than half the time or lessening* = 1 *Depressed more than half the time or worsening* = 2	0 1 2	RP focused on coping with depressed moods; simple CBT-informed advice for very mild depression	Refer to mental health treatment if sustained depressed mood.
How often were you in situations identified as being high risk for relapse? *Prompt for situations identified at orientation or prior call.*	*No people, places, and things* = 0 *1–2 encounters/week* = 1 *More than twice/week* = 2	0 1 2	Encourage avoidance and proactive coping efforts.	If housing or employment present chronic high risk, refer to housing or vocational services as needed.
Risk total		0–10		

Protective factors: high score = more protection			
How often have you done things with people who are sober or who do not have an alcohol/drug problem? *Prompt for social/leisure activities selected at orientation and/or prior call.*	*At least three times/week = 2* *1–2 times/week = 1* *None = 0*	0 1 2	Increase focus on positive activities if low, especially as patient becomes more stable.	Assist patient in identifying relevant activities: family, church, community, hobbies.
What have you done to pursue your personal goals? *Prompt for longer term and shorter term goals identified at orientation or in prior calls. Includes health-related goals.*	*Meaningful activity toward goal = 2* *Limited activity toward goal, or fulfilled "maintenance" goal = 1* *No activity toward goal or no goal = 0*	0 1 2	Increase focus on goals if low, especially as patient becomes more stable.	Assist patient in identifying services relevant to educational, vocational, or other goal.
Protective total		0–10		

Note. RP = relapse prevention; IOP = intensive outpatient program; CBT = cognitive–behavioral therapy.

having you come in for a face-to-face meeting so we have more time to address what's going on.

4. Review progress/goals since last call.

The counselor should ask the patient how he did with respect to the issues identified in the previous call. If a high-risk situation was anticipated and planned for, how did it go? Did the patient complete his prorecovery goals? The counselor can engage the patient in a detailed description of his successes. What did he feel good about? What was more difficult? The goals of this exercise include helping the patient recognize the inherently rewarding aspects of his abstinent lifestyle and troubleshoot difficult situations or change plans that are not working well.

5. Identify upcoming high-risk situations.

The counselor next asks the patient to think ahead to the interval until the next phone call. What situations might he encounter that could increase risk of relapse?

> You've had some cravings whenever you have been around your brother-in-law. Will you be seeing him in the next week?

> You will be stepping down to a lower level of care at your treatment program. That's a great milestone, but sometimes people find it is harder to stay abstinent when they have less support. What do you think?

The patient may or may not identify anything. If the patient has trouble anticipating high-risk situations yet reports having encountered them on a regular basis or reports continued cravings, the counselor can help him to see the connection between past difficult situations and the possibility that those same situations may arise in the foreseeable future. Some patients simply need help with learning to think about what they are going to be doing in the upcoming week and whether any of those plans entails some risk. CBT techniques, including functional analysis of prior relapses, can be helpful here.

6. Select target(s) for the remainder of the call.

Once the progress assessment and these other elements are completed, there will only be a limited amount of time for counseling (e.g., 10–20 minutes, depending on the planned duration of the call) before it is time to wrap up and schedule the next call. The patient and counselor should together choose one or two things on which to focus. These may include follow-up on patient's goals from the prior session, problem solving regarding newly identified or especially troublesome risks, and other pressing matters the patient may see as having a bearing on her ability to remain abstinent. This brief process will be an exercise in prioritizing for patient and counselor alike.

> Your goals were to attend AA daily and talk with your doctor about problems you've been having with your Zoloft. You made it to AA, but

you're still having trouble taking your meds. Bad moods are still a problem for you and may be a high-risk situation for you in the upcoming week. Which of these things should we focus on? Is there something even more important for your recovery right now?

If compliance with the call schedule is currently a problem, this is a good time to get it on the agenda.

7. Brief problem solving regarding target concern(s).

Once a specific target is identified, the counselor should engage the patient in problem solving. As much as possible, the counselor should guide the patient through the steps of problem solving rather than attempt to solve the problem for her by encouraging the patient to generate a few solutions and select one for implementation. The counselor can provide information and advice as needed but should avoid telling the patient what to do or getting into an unproductive back-and-forth in which she offers helpful suggestions and the patient rejects them. The counselor should avoid argumentation by responding reflectively to resistance and quickly getting back to the task at hand.

When motivation is flagging, this may be a signal that the patient is minimizing negative consequences of substance use and benefits of abstinence. The counselor can review the information gathered in the initial face-to-face session to help identify reasons for staying alcohol- and drug-free and inquire about the patient's current thoughts on the topic. The counselor can engage the patient in a discussion of the benefits of abstinence and how the patient can gain even more benefit from sober living. Motivational interviewing techniques (Miller & Rollnick, 2002) are particularly helpful in such situations.

As discussed earlier in this appendix, we make use of CBT techniques to help the patient develop better coping responses to anticipated high-risk situations or to other problems that have been selected to be addressed in the intervening interval before the next call. We tend to focus more on specific behavioral techniques to improve coping, rather than on techniques to alter biased cognitions. For example, we often do brief role-plays with patients so that they get a chance to practice a new behavior while still on the telephone. However, a patient's biased or otherwise inaccurate cognitions and beliefs that are getting in the way of her trying new coping behaviors or otherwise clearly sabotaging her recovery should be addressed.

In addition, there are many opportunities for the counselor to help the patient integrate her various recovery supports by shaping the patient's goals in a way that models such integration. One example might be connecting the patient's identified interpersonal relationship goals to people at church or meetings or work:

Is that something you could talk with your pastor about?

What about asking your brother to go with you to that appointment?

When you meet with your sponsor this week, could you ask for feedback about this?

8. Set goal(s) for interval before next call.

The patient should be reassured that he does not have to come up with lengthy or complicated tasks and goals. In fact, simple and brief is better, as long as specifics are provided. The counselor can help patients choose goals and tasks that are concrete and doable. It is better for the patient to experience success at a modest goal than to fail at a more ambitious one.

> Now let's go over what you'll be doing in the coming week, between now and our next telephone call. Given how things are going, what do you think the one or two most important goals should be for next week? The best kind of goal is one that is stated very clearly, so next week you'll be able to see if you've made progress on it. . . .
>
> Good. Now that you picked increasing your attendance at AA as your main goal for the week, what are the things you will do to reach that goal? The more specific you can be, the better. For example, rather than saying, "I'll go to AA," clarify how many meetings you plan to go to, where they are, and when they are. By doing that now, you'll have developed a good plan for the coming week.

9. Schedule the next phone call.

The call should end with scheduling the next phone call. If compliance has been a problem, the counselor should make sure the patient agrees that the designated time will work for him. If necessary, the patient and counselor can engage in brief problem solving regarding compliance with phone calls. If compliance has been a major issue, it should have been addressed earlier in the session, and can be reviewed at this point.

ADAPTIVE ALGORITHMS FOR STEPPED CARE

There are several possible approaches to devising an adaptive algorithm to adjust level of care on the basis of the patient's progress or the lack thereof. For example, counselors can be told to use their own clinical judgment and to recommend changes when they think it is advisable, or, counselors can be given general guidelines for stepped care, and urged to make use of them as they see fit. We have tried to provide more formal algorithms to counselors that make use of data collected in the progress assessment at the beginning of each call.

In the algorithm we developed first, patients who reported any recent use or extreme concern about their ability to remain abstinent for the next week were automatically placed in the *high-risk* category. However, patients could also be placed in the high-risk category by virtue of at least moderately concerning responses on most of the other risk items, coupled with low scores on the protective factors. The *low-risk* category, in contrast, required low scores on all risk items plus at least some evidence of prorecovery behaviors and activities. Patients who did not end up in either high- or low-risk categories were placed by default in the *moderate-risk* category. This system had predictive validity, but it was difficult to use.

Therefore, in our current study with cocaine patients, we have developed a simpler and more straightforward algorithm, which is keyed on changes in the balance between risk and protective scores and also takes into account current status in IOP or OP treatment that the patient may still be participating in.

1. If the patient shows an increased risk factors score, a decreased protective factors score, or both, and it combines to an overall shift of 4 points in the wrong direction, the clinician should attempt to address it with the patient in a more comprehensive fashion during the call. It would be appropriate to have a longer than usual call to address the recent change and help the patient develop a plan to decrease risk-related behaviors, increase protective behaviors, or both. If the patient can agree to a reasonable plan and is confident in his or her ability to remain abstinent, then the next call will be scheduled as usual.

2. If the patient cannot agree to a reasonable plan or is concerned about using alcohol or drugs, or if the worrisome negative overall shift in risk and protective factors scores is maintained at the next call, then the counselor should (a) encourage the patient to make use of treatment if the patient is still meaningfully engaged in IOP or OP or (b) increase the frequency of contacts immediately, if the patient is not engaged in IOP or OP.

3. The usual starting point for increased frequency of contacts would be a scheduled call at half the usual interval (e.g., if the patient has been calling every 2 weeks, offer a call at 1 week) with the availability of emergency calls sooner if needed. If the patient is not confident she can remain alcohol- and drug-free for that time period, then the counselor should decrease the interval by half again and consider a face-to-face session (discussed later). If the patient can follow through on her plans, then the counselor can continue with increased call frequency until the risk–protection balance shifts back to a more healthy ratio.

4. The counselor should offer a face-to-face evaluation session if

(a) the patient expresses low confidence in ability to remain abstinent for at least 1 week, (b) the patient has difficulty following through on plans to lower risk and increase protection with phone contact, or (c) the nature of the patient's problem requires case management that is too cumbersome to perform over the phone.

Face-to-Face Evaluation Sessions

By the time an in-person session is scheduled, the counselor may have already spent several phone calls "putting out fires" with a patient who is experiencing one or more crises or who is showing minimal compliance or flagging motivation. The goal of the session is to take a step back from the immediate situation and get a broader assessment of what is going on. The evaluation session should include a detailed debriefing of any relapse episodes and also address motivation and commitment to change in a more general sense.

When the patient has a slip or becomes at high risk of relapse despite ongoing phone intervention, it may be that the focus of sessions and the between-session goals are not quite on target with respect to the patient's true relapse risks, in which case the general thrust of problem-solving efforts needs to be revised. Examples would be patients who have misidentified their most important risky situations to follow on an ongoing basis or patients who do not have adequate coping skills to deal with unavoidable risky situations. Patients whose case management needs are not being met would also fall in this category.

Another possibility is that the patient's motivation to achieve or maintain abstinence is failing and the benefits of recovery do not seem to be sufficiently rewarding to counteract the lure of alcohol or drug use. Asking the patient to rate how important abstinence is to her and how confident she is that she can achieve or maintain it will, with appropriate follow-up questions, helps the counselor to determine where to focus the rest of the session.

We follow this basic outline for face-to-face evaluation sessions, which makes use of the general principles as well as specific active components of motivational interviewing (Miller & Rollnick, 2002):

1. Set an agenda and acknowledge the patient for coming in to address current problems.
2. Go over any episodes of use, with emphasis on triggers for the relapse. Did the patient mount any coping behaviors, and if so, why does she think they were not effective?
3. Assess current motivation for being alcohol- and drug-free using scales to assess the importance of abstinence and confidence in being able to cope without using.

4. If patient attaches low importance to being abstinent, (a) acknowledge difficulty of following through on action plans when feeling low motivation, (b) use patient's response to "What would it take to increase importance?" to find hooks for increasing motivation, and/or (c) develop a homework task to address motivation.
5. If perceived importance of abstinence is high but confidence is low, (a) explore past and present efforts at change to find what has worked in the past and what is different now and (b) use the patient's response to "What would it take to increase confidence?" to guide problem-solving efforts.

Further Therapeutic Options on the Stepped-Care Ladder

If the face-to-face evaluation session raises further alarm bells, or if the clinically significant shift in the balance of risk and protective factors does not reverse itself relatively quickly, our algorithm calls for the implementation of further face-to-face treatment. We offer individual CBT sessions (1–2/week) for up to 8 weeks to patients in this situation, or we help the patient reengage with a local community IOP or OP program if the patient prefers. In cases in which the patient has been engaged in a considerable amount of heavy drinking over an extended period, the possible need for formal detoxification also should be considered.

Lateral Adaptations and Case Management Referrals

In addition to *vertical* moves through stepped care, the protocol provides guidance on when to consider what might be called *lateral* moves. In these situations, the patient stays at the same level and frequency of contact, but the content of the intervention is modified. For example, decreases in self-efficacy might be addressed by rehearsing coping responses during the call and suggesting further confidence-building exercises between calls. Similarly, increases in depressive symptoms could be addressed by using CBT techniques that challenge cognitions and attributions associated with depression. These procedures qualify as adaptive treatment, as long as "if–then" statements are used to link specific scores on assessment items or measures to specific modifications in treatment. Recommendations for lateral adaptations and case management efforts are illustrated in sample items from the progress assessment in Table A.1.

MAXIMIZING ADHERENCE TO TELEPHONE CONTINUING CARE

As discussed earlier, it is crucial for the clinician and patient to arrive at a calling plan during the orientation, particularly with regard to who should call whom and when. When a call is missed (i.e., either the patient does not call in or the clinician calls and there is no answer), it is the clinician's responsibility to try to reach the patient, determine the reason for the missed appointment, and reengage the patient in regular phone session attendance. The clinician should make active efforts to reengage a missing patient for up to 1 month after a missed session, including phone calls to the patient, phone calls to support people, and letters to the patient. After a month from the last contact, the patient is considered inactive in treatment but may return at any point during the treatment window (this will, of course, vary, depending on staffing and other resources).

FINAL REMARKS

The material provided in this appendix can serve as a blueprint for the provision of TEL, with or without adaptive components, for patients with substance use disorders. Although we have empirical evidence that these procedures are effective—with regard to both retaining patients and yielding good outcomes—we are still very early on in the process of developing and evaluating such interventions. Therefore, clinicians and programs that are interesting in implementing these procedures should make sure that they are compatible with the rest of their programming. Each clinic presents its own set of challenges, and our protocol and procedures will likely need some modification to work effectively in other environments. In the spirit of adaptive treatment, programs should carefully document the initial modifications that are made to improve implementation and results and any subsequent modifications to address additional problems that surface after the continuing care protocol has been in use for a time.

REFERENCES

ALLHAT Collaborative Research Group. (2002). Major outcomes in high-risk hypertensive patients randomized to angiotensin-converting enzyme inhibitor or calcium channel blocker vs. diuretic: The Antihypertensive and Lipid-Lowering Treatment to Prevent Heart Attack Trial. *JAMA, 288,* 2981–2997.

Alterman, A. I., Kampman, K., Boardman, C. R., Cacciola, J. S., Rutherford, M. R., McKay, J. R., & Maany, I. (1997). A cocaine-positive baseline urine predicts outpatient treatment attrition and failure to attain initial abstinence. *Drug and Alcohol Dependence, 46,* 79–85.

American Psychiatric Association. (1994). *Diagnostic and statistical manual of mental disorders* (4th ed.). Washington, DC: Author.

American Society of Addiction Medicine. (2001). *ASAM PPC–2R-ASAM Patient Placement Criteria for the Treatment of Substance-Related Disorders* (2nd ed., rev.). Chevy Chase, MD: Author.

Andersen, R. M. (1995). Revisiting the behavioral model and access to medical care: Does it matter? *Journal of Health and Social Behavior, 36,* 1–10.

Anderson, D. J., McGovern, J. P., & Dupont, R. L. (1999). The origins of the Minnesota Model of addiction treatment: A first person account. *Journal of Addictive Diseases, 18,* 107–114.

Anglin, M. D., Hser, Y.-I., & Grella, C. E. (1997). Drug addiction and treatment careers among clients in the Drug Abuse Treatment Outcome Study (DATOS). *Psychology of Addictive Behavior, 11,* 308–323.

Annis, H. M., & Davis, C. S. (1989). Relapse prevention. In R. K. Hester & W. R. Miller (Eds.), *Handbook of alcoholism treatment approaches* (pp. 170–182). New York: Pergamon Press.

Anton, R. F., O'Malley, S. S., Ciraulo, D. A., Cisler, R. A., Couper, D., Donovan, D. M., et al. (2006). Combined pharmacotherapies and behavioral interventions for alcohol dependence. *JAMA, 295,* 2003–2017.

Anton, R. F., Oroszi, G., O'Malley, S., Couper, D., Swift, R., Pettinati, H., et al. (2008). An evaluation of mu-opioid receptor (OPRM1) as a predictor of naltrexone response in the treatment of alcohol dependence: Results from the COMBINE study. *Archives of General Psychiatry, 65,* 135–144.

Appel, P. W., Ellison, A. A., Jansky, H. K., & Oldak, R. (2004). Barriers to enrollment in drug abuse treatment and suggestions for reducing them: Opinions of drug injecting street outreach clients and other system stakeholders. *American Journal of Drug and Alcohol Abuse, 30,* 129–153.

Babor, T. F., & Grant, M. (Eds.). (1992). Project on identification and management of alcohol-related problems. *Report of Phase II: A randomized clinical trial of brief interventions in primary health care.* Geneva, Switzerland: World Health Organization.

Bandura, A. (1991). Social cognitive theory of self-regulation. *Organizational Behavior and Human Decision Processes, 50,* 248–287.

Baron, R. M., & Kenny, D. A. (1986). The moderator-mediator variable distinction in social psychological research: Conceptual, strategic, and statistical considerations. *Journal of Personality and Social Psychology, 51*, 1173–1182.

Baskin, T. W., Tierney, S. C., Minami, T., & Wampold, B. E. (2003). Establishing specificity in psychotherapy: A meta-analysis of structural equivalence of placebo controls. *Journal of Consulting and Clinical Psychology, 71*, 973–979.

Bauer, L. O., Covault, J., Harel, O., Das, S., Gelernter, J., Anton, R., et al. (2007). Variation in GABRA2 predicts drinking behavior in Project MATCH subjects. *Alcoholism: Clinical and Experimental Research, 31*, 1780–1787.

Beck, A. T., Rush, A. J., Shaw, B. F., & Emery, G. (1979). *Cognitive therapy of depression*. New York: Guilford Press.

Bennett, G. A., Withers, J., Thomas, P. W., Higgins, D. S., Bailey, J., Parry, L., et al. (2005). A randomized trial of early warning signs relapse prevention training in the treatment of alcohol dependence. *Addictive Behaviors, 30*, 1111–1124.

Bickel, W. K., & Marsch, L. A. (2007). A future for the prevention and treatment of drug abuse: Applications of computer-based interactive technology. In J. E. Henningfield, P. B. Santora, & W. K. Bickel (Eds.), *Addiction treatment: Science and policy for the twenty-first century* (pp. 35–44). Baltimore: Johns Hopkins University Press.

Bickel, W. K., Marsch, L. A., Buchhalter, A. R., & Badger, G. J. (2008). Computerized behavior therapy for opioid-dependent outpatients: A randomized controlled trial. *Experimental and Clinical Psychopharmacology, 16*, 132–143.

Bischof, G., Grothues, J. M., Reinhardt, S., Meyer, C., John, U., & Rumpf, H.-J. (2008). Evaluation of a telephone-based stepped care intervention for alcohol-related disorders: A randomized clinical trial. *Drug and Alcohol Dependence, 93*, 244–251.

Bourgois, P., Martinez, A., Kral, A., Edlin, B. R., Schonberg, J., & Ciccarone, D. (2006). Reinterpreting ethnic patterns among white and African-American men who inject heroin: A social science of medicine approach. *Public Library of Science Medicine, 3*, 0001–0011.

Breslin, F. C., Sobell, M. B., Sobell, L. C., Buchan, G., & Cunningham, J. A. (1997). Toward a stepped care approach to treating problem drinkers: The predictive utility of within-treatment variables and therapist prognostic ratings. *Addiction, 92*, 1479–1489.

Breslin, F. C., Sobell, M. B., Sobell, L. C., Cunningham, J. A., Sdao-Jarvie, K., & Borsoi, D. (1999). Problem drinkers: Evaluation of a stepped-care approach. *Journal of Substance Abuse, 10*, 217–232.

Brooner, R. K., & Kidorf, M. S. (2002). Using behavioral reinforcement to improve methadone treatment participation. *Science and Practice Perspective, 1*, 38–46.

Brooner, R. K., Kidorf, M. S., King, V. L., Stoller, K. B., Neufeld, K. J., & Kolodner, K. (2007). Comparing adaptive stepped care and monetary-based voucher interventions for opioid dependence. *Drug & Alcohol Dependence, 88*(Suppl. 2), S14–S23.

Brooner, R. K., Kidorf, M. S., King, V. L., Stoller, K. B., Peirce, J. M., Bigelow, G. E., et al. (2004). Behavioral contingencies improve counseling attendance in an adaptive treatment model. *Journal of Substance Abuse Treatment, 27*, 223–232.

Brown, B. S., O'Grady, K., Battjes, R. J., & Farrell, E. V. (2004). Factors associated with treatment outcomes in an aftercare population. *The American Journal on Addiction, 13*, 447–460.

Brown, T., Seraganian, P., Tremblay, J., & Annis, H. (2002). Process and outcome changes with relapse prevention versus 12-step aftercare programs for substance abusers. *Addiction, 97*, 677–689.

Brownell, K. D., Marlatt, G. A., Lichtenstein, E., & Wilson, G. T. (1986). Understanding and preventing relapse. *American Psychologist, 41*, 765–782.

Buhringer, G. (2006). Allocating treatment options to patient profiles: Clinical art or science? *Addiction, 101*, 646–652.

Burke, B. L., Arkowitz, H., & Menchola, M. (2003). The efficacy of motivational interviewing: A meta-analysis of controlled clinical trials. *Journal of Consulting and Clinical Psychology, 71*, 843–861.

Butler, C., Rollnick, S., Cohen, D., Bachman, M., Russell, I., & Stott, N. (1999). Motivational consulting versus brief advice for smokers in general practice: A randomized trial. *British Journal of General Practice, 49*, 611–616.

Cacciola, J. S., Camilleri, A. C., Carise, D., Rikoon, S. H., McKay, J. R., McLellan, A. T., et al. (2008). Extending residential care through telephone counseling: Initial results from the Betty Ford Center Focused Continuing Care Protocol. *Addictive Behaviors, 33*, 1208–1216.

Carels, R. A., Darby, L., Cacciapaglia, H. M., Douglass, O. M., Harper, J., Kaplar, M. E., et al. (2005). Applying a stepped-care approach to the treatment of obesity. *Journal of Psychosomatic Research, 59*, 375–383.

Carmen, B., Angeles, M., Ana, M., & Maria, A. J. (2004). Efficacy and safety of naltrexone and acamprosate in the treatment of alcohol dependence: A systematic review. *Addiction, 99*, 811–828.

Carroll, K. M. (1998). *A cognitive–behavioral approach: Treating cocaine addiction* (NIH Publication No. 98-4308). Rockville, MD: National Institute on Drug Abuse.

Carroll, K. M., Ball, S. A., Martino, S., Nich, C., Babuscio, T., Nuro, K., et al. (2008). Computer-assisted delivery of cognitive–behavioral therapy for addiction: A randomized trial of CBT4CBT. *The American Journal of Psychiatry, 165*, 881–888.

Carroll, K. M., Fenton, L., Ball, S. A., Nich, C., Frankforter, T., Shi, J., et al. (2004). Efficacy of disulfiram and cognitive behavior therapy in cocaine-dependent outpatients: A randomized placebo-controlled trial. *Archives of General Psychiatry, 61*, 264–272.

Carroll, K. M., Nich, C., Ball, S. A., McCance, E., & Rounsaville, B. (1998). Treatment of cocaine and alcohol dependence with psychotherapy and disulfiram. *Addiction, 93*, 713–728.

Carroll, K. M., Nich, C., & Rounsaville, B. J. (1995). Differential symptom reduction in depressed cocaine abusers treated with psychotherapy and pharmacotherapy. *Journal of Nervous and Mental Disease, 183*, 251–259.

Carroll, K. M., Rounsaville, B. J., & Gawin, F. H. (1991). A comparative trial of psychotherapies for ambulatory cocaine abusers: Relapse prevention and interpersonal psychotherapy. *American Journal of Drug and Alcohol Abuse, 17,* 229–247.

Carroll, K. M., Rounsaville, B. J., Nich, C., Gordon, L. T., Wirtz, P. W., & Gawin, F. (1994). One-year follow-up of psychotherapy and pharmacotherapy for cocaine dependence: Delayed emergence of psychotherapy effects. *Archives of General Psychiatry, 51,* 989–997.

Chen, S., Barnett, P. G., Sempel, J. M., & Timko, C. (2006). Outcomes and costs of matching the intensity of dual-diagnosis treatment to patients' symptom severity. *Journal of Substance Abuse Treatment, 31,* 95–105.

Childress, A. R., Ehrman, R. N., Wang, Z., Li, Y., Sciortino, N., Hukun, J., Jens, W., et al. (2008). Prelude to passion: Limbic activation by "unseen" drug and sexual cues. *PLoS ONE, 3*(1), 1–6. doi: 10.1371/journal.pone.0001506

Chutuape, M. A., Katz, E. C., & Stitzer, M. L. (2001). Methods for enhancing transition of substance dependent patients from inpatient to outpatient treatment. *Drug and Alcohol Dependence, 61,* 137–143.

Clark, M. A., Rakowski, W., Ehrich, B., Rimer, B. K., Velicer, W. F., Dube, C. E., et al. (2002). The effect of a stage-matched and tailored intervention on repeat mammography. *American Journal of Preventive Medicine, 22,* 1–7.

Cohen, J. (1988). *Statistical power analysis for the behavioral sciences.* Hillsdale, NJ: Erlbaum.

Collins, L. M., Murphy, S. A., & Bierman, K. L. (2004). A conceptual framework for adaptive preventive interventions. *Prevention Science, 5,* 185–196.

Collins, L. M., Murphy, S. A., Nair, V. N., & Strecher, V. J. (2005). A strategy for optimizing and evaluating behavioral interventions. *Annals of Behavioral Medicine, 30,* 65–68.

Collins, L. M., Murphy, S. A., & Strecher, V. (2007). The multiphase optimization strategy (MOST) and the sequential multiple assignment randomized trial (SMART): New methods for more potent eHealth interventions. *American Journal of Preventive Medicine, 32,* S112–S118.

Collins, R. L., Kashdan, T. B., & Gollnisch, G. (2003). The feasibility of using cellular phones to collect ecological momentary assessment data: Application to alcohol consumption. *Experimental and Clinical Psychopharmacology, 11,* 73–78.

Connecticut Department of Mental Health and Addiction Services. (2006). *Practice guidelines for recovery-oriented behavioral health care.* Hartford, CT: Author.

Connecticut Department of Mental Health and Addiction Services. (2007, October 4). *Information.* Hartford, CT: Author.

Connors, G. J., Carroll, K. M., DiClemente, C. C., Longabaugh, R., & Donovan, D. M. (1997). The therapeutic alliance and its relationship to alcoholism treatment participation and outcome. *Journal of Consulting and Clinical Psychology, 65,* 588–598.

Connors, G. J., Maisto, S. A., & Zywiak, W. H. (1996). Understanding relapse in the broader context of post-treatment functioning. *Addiction, 91*(Suppl.), S173–S190.

Connors, G. J., Tarbox, A. R., & Faillace, L. A. (1992). Achieving and maintaining gains among problem drinkers: Process and outcome results. *Behavior Therapy, 23,* 449–474.

Cooney, N. L., Kadden, R. M., Litt, M. D., & Getter, H. (1991). Matching alcoholics to coping skills or interactional therapies: Two-year follow-up results. *Journal of Consulting and Clinical Psychology, 59,* 598–601.

Coviello, D. M., Zanis, D. A., Wesnoski, S. A., & Alterman, A. I. (2006). The effectiveness of outreach case management in re-enrolling discharged methadone patients. *Drug and Alcohol Dependence, 85,* 56–65.

Crews, F. T., Braun, C. J., Hoplight, B., Switzer, R. C., III, & Knapp, D. J. (2000). Binge ethanol consumption causes differential brain damage in young adolescent rats compared with adult rats. *Alcoholism: Clinical and Experimental Research, 24,* 1712–1723.

Crews, F. T., Buckley, T., Dodd, P. R., Ende, G., Foley, N., Harper, C., et al. (2005). Alcoholic neurobiology: Changes in dependence and recovery. *Alcoholism: Clinical and Experimental Research, 29,* 1504–1513.

Crits-Christoph, P., Siqueland, L., Blaine, J., Frank, A., Luborsky, L., Onken, L. S., et al. (1999). Psychosocial treatments for cocaine dependence: National Institute on Drug Abuse Collaborative Cocaine Treatment Study. *Archives of General Psychiatry, 56,* 493–502.

Cunningham, J. A., Sobell, L. C., Sobell, M. B., Agrawal, S., & Toneatto, T. (1993). Barriers to treatment: Why alcoholics and drug abusers delay or never seek treatment. *Addictive Behaviors, 18,* 347–353.

Dackis, C. A., Kampman, K. M., Lynch, K. G., Pettinati, H. M., & O'Brien, C. P. (2005). A double-blind, placebo-controlled trial of modafinil for cocaine dependence. *Neuropsychopharmacology, 30,* 205–11.

Davidson, L., O'Connell, M. J., Tondora, J., Lawless, M., & Evans, A. C. (2005). Recovery in serious mental illness: A new wine or just a new bottle? *Professional Psychology: Research and Practice, 36,* 480–487.

Dennis, M. L., Foss, M. A., & Scott, C. K. (2007). An eight-year perspective on the relationship between the duration of abstinence and other aspects of recovery. *Evaluation Review, 31,* 585–612.

Dennis, M. L., & Scott, C. K. (2007, December). Managing addiction as a chronic condition. *Addiction Science and Clinical Practice,* 45–55.

Dennis, M. L., Scott, C. K., & Funk, R. (2003). An experimental evaluation of recovery management checkups (RMC) for people with chronic substance use disorders. *Evaluation and Program Planning, 26,* 339–352.

DeRubeis, R. J., Brotman, M. A., & Gibbons, C. J. (2005). A conceptual and methodological analysis of the nonspecifics argument. *Clinical Psychology: Science and Practice, 12,* 174–183.

DiClemente, C. C. (2003). *Addiction and change: How addictions develop and addicted people recover.* New York: Guilford Press.

Domino, K. B., Hornbein, T. F., Polissar, N. L., Renner, G., Johnson, J., Alberti, S., & Hankes, L. (2005). Risk factors for relapse in health care professionals with substance use disorders. *JAMA, 293,* 1453–1460.

Donovan, D. M. (1996). Assessment issues and domains in the prediction of relapse. *Addiction, 91*, 29–36.

Dunn, C., Deroo, L., & Rivara, F. P. (2001). The use of brief interventions adapted from motivational interviewing across behavioral domains: A systematic review. *Addiction, 96*, 1725–1742.

DuPont, R. L., McLellan, A. T., White, W. L., Merlo, L. J., & Gold, M. S. (2009). Setting the standard for recovery: Physicians' Health Programs. *Journal of Substance Abuse Treatment, 36*, 159–171.

Dwight-Johnson, M., Sherbourne, C. D., Liao, D., & Wells, K. B. (2000). Treatment preferences among depressed primary care patients. *Journal of General Internal Medicine, 15*, 527–534.

Elman, I., Lukas, S. E., Karlsgodt, K. H., Gasic, G. P., & Breiter, H. C. (2003). Acute cortisol administration triggers craving in individuals with cocaine dependence. *Psychopharmacological Bulletin, 37*, 84–89.

Epstein, E. E., & McCrady, B. S. (1998). Behavioral couples treatment of alcohol and drug use disorders: Current status and innovations. *Clinical Psychology Review, 18*, 689–711.

Fava, M., Rush, A. J., Wisniewski, S. R., Nierenberg, A. A., Alpert, J. E., McGrath, P. J., et al. (STAR*D StudyTeam). (2006). A comparison of mirtazapine and nortriptyline following two consecutive failed medication treatments for depressed outpatients: A STAR*D report. *The American Journal of Psychiatry, 163*, 1161–1172.

Febbraro, G. A. R., & Clum, G. A. (1998). Meta-analytic investigation of the effectiveness of self-regulatory components in the treatment of adult problem behaviors. *Clinical Psychology Review, 18*, 143–161.

Festinger, D. S., Marlowe, D. B., Lee, P. A., Kirby, K. C., Bovasso, G., & McLellan, A. T. (2002). Status hearings in drug court: When more is less and less is more. *Drug & Alcohol Dependence, 68*, 151–157.

Fiorentine, R. (1998). Effective drug treatment: Testing the distal needs hypothesis. *Journal of Substance Abuse Treatment, 15*, 281–289.

Fleming, M. F., Barry, K. L., Manwell, L. B., Johnson, K., & London, R. (1997). Brief physician advice for problem alcohol drinkers: A randomized controlled trial in community-based primary care practices. *JAMA, 277*, 1039–1045.

Fletcher, A. M. (2001). *Sober for good*. Boston: Houghton Mifflin.

Foote, A., & Erfurt, J. C. (1991). Effects of EAP follow-up on prevention of relapse among substance abuse clients. *Journal of Studies on Alcohol, 52*, 241–248.

Forman, R. F. (2002). One AA meeting doesn't fit all: 6 keys to prescribing 12-step programs. *Psychiatry Online, 1*, 1–6.

Fowler, J. S., Volkow, N. D., Kassed, C. A., & Chang, L. (2007, April). Imaging the addicted brain. *Science & Practice Perspectives*, 4–19.

Franklin, T. R., Acton, P. D., Maldjian, J. A., Gray, J. D., Croft, J. R., Dackis, C. A., et al. (2002). Decreased gray matter concentration in the insular, orbitofrontal, cingulated, and temporal cortices of cocaine patients. *Biological Psychiatry, 51*, 134–142.

Franklin, T. R., Lohoff, F. W., Wang, Z., Sciortino, N., Harper, D., Li, Y., et al. (2008). DAT genotype modulates brain and behavioral responses elicited by cigarette cues. *Neuropsychopharmacology, 34*, 717–728.

Friedmann, P. D., Hendrickson, J. C., Gerstein, D. R., & Zhang, Z. (2004). The effect of matching comprehensive services to patients' needs on drug use improvement in addiction treatment. *Addiction, 99*, 962–972.

Garbutt, J. C., Kranzler, H. R., O'Malley, S. S., Gastfriend, D. R., Pettinati, H. M., Silverman, B. L., et al. (2005). Efficacy and tolerability of long-acting injectable naltrexone for alcohol dependence: A randomized controlled trial. *JAMA, 293*, 1617–1625.

Gilbert, F. S. (1988). The effect of type of aftercare follow-up on treatment outcome among alcoholics. *Journal of Studies on Alchohol, 49*, 149–159.

Godley, M. D., Garner, B. R., Funk, R. R., Passetti, L. L., & Godley, S. H. (2008, June–July). *A validity study of the Washington Circle continuity of care performance measure*. Paper presented at the Research Society on Alcoholism Conference, Washington, DC.

Godley, M. D., Godley, S. H., Dennis, M. L., Funk, R. R., & Passetti, L. L. (2006). The effect of assertive continuing care on continuing care linkage, adherence, and abstinence following residential treatment for adolescents with substance use disorders. *Addiction, 102*, 81–93.

Godley, S. H., Godley, M. D., Karvinen, T., & Slown, L. L. (2001). *The assertive aftercare protocol: A case manager's manual for working with adolescents after residential treatment of alcohol and other substance use disorders*. Bloomington, IL: Lighthouse Institute.

Goldman, D., Oroszi, G., & Ducci, F. (2005). The genetics of addictions: Uncovering the genes. *Nature Reviews Genetics, 6*, 521–532.

Gorski, T. (1995). *Relapse prevention therapy workbook: Managing core personality and lifestyle issues*. Independence, MO: Herald House.

Graham, K., Annis, H. M., Brett, P. J., & Venesoen, P. (1996). A controlled field trial of group versus individual cognitive–behavioral training for relapse prevention. *Addiction, 91*, 1127–1139.

Grant, B. F. (1997). Barriers to alcoholism treatment: Reasons for not seeking treatment in a general population sample. *Journal of Studies on Alcohol, 58*, 365–371.

Grant, B. F., Stinson, F. S., Dawson, D. A., Chou, S. P., Dufour, M. C., Compton, W., et al. (2004). Prevalence and co-occurrence of substance use disorders and independent mood and anxiety disorders: Results from the National Epidemiologic Survey on Alcohol and Related Conditions. *Archives of General Psychiatry, 61*, 807–816.

Gueorguieva, R., Wu, R., Pittman, B., Cramer, J., Rosenheck, R. A., O'Malley, S. S., et al. (2007). New insights into the efficacy of naltrexone based on trajectory-based reanalyses of two negative clinical trials. *Biological Psychiatry, 61*, 1290–1295.

Gustafson, D. H., Palesh, T. E., Picard, R. W., Plsek, P. E., Maher, L., & Capoccia, V. A. (2005). Automating addiction treatment: Enhancing the human experience and creating a fix for the future. In R. Bushko (Ed.), *Future of intelligent and extelligent health environment* (pp. 186–206). Amsterdam: IOS Press.

Hall, M. J., & Tidwell, W. C. (2003). Internet recovery for substance abuse and alcoholism: An exploratory study of service users. *Journal of Substance Abuse Treatment, 24*, 161–167.

Hall, S. M., Havassy, B. E., & Wasserman, D. A. (1991). Effects of commitment to abstinence, positive moods, stress, and coping on relapse to cocaine use. *Journal of Consulting and Clinical Psychology, 59*, 526–532.

Hall, S. M., Humfleet, G. L., Reus, V. I., Munoz, R. F., & Cullen, J. (2004). Extended nortriptyline and psychological treatment for cigarette smoking. *The American Journal of Psychiatry, 161*, 2100–2107.

Hammersley, R. (1994). A digest of memory phenomena for addiction research. *Addiction, 89*, 283–293.

Harris, A. H. S., Humphreys, K., Bowe, T., Kivlahan, D. R., & Finney, J. W. (in press). Measuring the quality of substance use disorder treatment: Evaluating the validity of the VA Continuity of Care Performance Measure. *Journal of Substance Abuse Treatment.*

Harris, A. H. S., McKellar, J. D., Moos, R. H., Schaefer, J. A., & Cronkite, R. C. (2006). Predictors of engagement in continuing care following residential substance use disorder treatment. *Drug and Alcohol Dependence, 84*, 93–101.

Hasin, D. S., Nunes, E., & Meydan, J. (2004). Comorbidity of alcohol, drug, and psychiatric disorders: Epidemiology. In H. R. Kranzler & J. A. Tinsley (Eds.), *Dual diagnosis and psychiatric treatment: Substance abuse and comorbid disorders* (2nd ed., pp. 1–34). New York: Marcel Dekker.

Havassy, B. E., Wasserman, D. A., & Hall, S. M. (1995). Social relationships and abstinence from cocaine in an American treatment sample. *Addiction, 90*, 699–710.

Hawkins, J. D., Catalano, R. F., Gillmore, M. R., & Wells, E. A. (1989). Skills training for drug abusers: Generalization, maintenance, and effects of drug use. *Journal of Consulting and Clinical Psychology, 57*, 559–563.

Heather, N. (1996). The public health and brief interventions for excessive alcohol consumption: The British experience. *Addictive Behavior, 21*, 857–868.

Helmus, T. C., Saules, K. K., Schoener, E. P., & Roll, J. M. (2003). Reinforcement of counseling attendance and alcohol abstinence in a community-based dual-diagnosis treatment program: A feasibility study. *Psychology of Addictive Behaviors, 17*, 249–251.

Helzer, J. E., Badger, G. J., Rose, G. L., Mongeon, J. A., & Searles, J. S. (2002). Decline in alcohol consumption during two years of daily reporting. *Journal of Studies on Alcohol, 63*, 551–558.

Higgins, S. T., Badger, G. J., & Budney, A. J. (2000). Initial abstinence and success in achieving longer term cocaine abstinence. *Experimental and Clinical Psychopharmacology, 8*, 377–386.

Higgins, S. T., Sigmon, S. C., Wong, C. J., Heil, S. H., Badger, G. J., Donham, R., et al. (2003). Community reinforcement therapy for cocaine-dependent outpatients. *Archives of General Psychiatry, 60,* 1043–1052.

Hitchock, H. C., Stainback, R. D., & Roque, G. M. (1995). Effects of halfway house placement on retention of patients in substance abuse aftercare. *American Journal of Drug and Alcohol Abuse, 21,* 379–390.

Horng, F., & Chueh, K. (2004). Effectiveness of telephone follow-up and counseling in aftercare for alcoholism. *Journal of Nursing Research, 12,* 11–19.

Howard, K. I., Moras, K., Brill, P., Martinovich, Z., & Lutz, W. (1996). Efficacy, effectiveness and patient progress. *American Psychologist, 51,* 1059–1064.

Hser, Y. I., Anglin, M. D., Grella, C., Longshore, D., & Prendergast, M. L. (1997). Drug treatment careers: A conceptual framework and existing research findings. *Journal of Substance Abuse Treatment, 14,* 543–558.

Hser, Y. I., Grella, C. E., Hsieh, S. C., Anglin, M. D., & Brown, B. S. (1999). Prior treatment experience related to process and outcomes in DATOS. *Drug and Alcohol Dependence, 57,* 137–150.

Hser, Y. I., Longshore, D., & Anglin, M. D. (2007). The life course perspective on drug use: A conceptual framework for understanding drug use trajectories. *Evaluation Review: A Journal of Applied Social Research, 31,* 515–547.

Hubbard, R. L., Leimberger, J. D., Haynes, L., Patkar, A. A., Holter, J., Liepman, M. R., et al. (2007). Telephone enhancement of long-term engagement (TELE) in continuing care for substance abuse treatment: A NIDA Clinical Trials Network study. *American Journal on Addictions, 16,* 495–502.

Hufford, M. R., Witkiewitz, K., Shields, A. L., Kodya, S., & Caruso, J. C. (2003). Applying nonlinear dynamics to the prediction of alcohol use disorder treatment outcome. *Journal of Abnormal Psychology, 112,* 219–227.

Humphreys, K. (2004). *Circles of recovery: Self-help organizations for addictions.* Cambridge, England: Cambridge University Press.

Humphreys, K., & Tucker, J. A. (2002). Toward more responsive and effective intervention systems for alcohol-related problems. *Addiction, 97,* 126–132.

Institute of Medicine. (2001). *Crossing the quality chasm: A new health system for the twenty-first century.* Washington, DC: National Academies Press.

Institute of Medicine. (2006). *Improving the quality of health care for mental and substance-use conditions: Quality chasm series.* Washington, DC: National Academies Press.

Ito, J. R., & Donovan, D. M. (1986). Aftercare in alcoholism treatment: A review. In W. R. Miller & N. Heather (Eds.), *The addictive behaviors: Processes of change* (pp. 435–456). New York: Plenum Press.

Ito, J. R., Donovan, D. M., & Hall, J. J. (1988). Relapse prevention in alcohol aftercare: Effects on drinking outcomes, change process, and aftercare attendance. *British Journal of Addiction, 83,* 171–181.

Jarrett, R. B., Kraft, D., Doyle, J., Foster, B. M., Eaves, G. G., & Silver, P. C. (2001). Preventing recurrent depression using cognitive therapy with and without a continuation phase. *Archives of General Psychiatry, 58,* 381–388.

Johnson, B. A., Roache, J. D., Javors, M. A., DiClemente, C. C., Cloninger, C. R., Prihoda, T. J., et al. (2000). Ondansetron for reduction of drinking among biologically predisposed alcoholic patients: A randomized controlled trial. *JAMA, 284,* 963–71.

Johnson, B. A., Rosenthal, N., Capece, J. A., Wiegand, F., Mao, L., Beyers, K., et al. (2007). Topiramate for treating alcohol dependence: A randomized controlled trial. *JAMA, 298,* 1641–1651.

Junghanns, K., Backhaus, J., Tietz, U., Lange, W., Bernzen, J., Wetterling, T., et al. (2003). Impaired serum cortisol stress response is a predictor of early relapse. *Alcohol and Alcoholism, 38,* 189–193.

Kadden, R. M., Litt, M. D., Cooney, N. L., Kabela, E., & Getter, H. (2001). Prospective matching of alcoholic clients to cognitive–behavioral or interactional group therapy. *Journal of Studies on Alcohol, 62,* 359–369.

Kakko, J., Gronbladh, L., Svanborg, K. D., von Wachenfeldt, J., Ruck, C., Rawlings, B., et al. (2007). A stepped care strategy using buprenorphine and methadone versus conventional methadone maintenance in heroin dependence: A randomized controlled trial. *The American Journal of Psychiatry, 164,* 797–803.

Kalivas, P. W. (2007). Neurobiology of cocaine addiction: Implications for new pharmacotherapy. *American Journal on Addictions, 16,* 71–78.

Karno, M. P., & Longabaugh, R. (2003). Patient depressive symptoms and therapist focus on emotional material: A new look at Project MATCH. *Journal of Studies on Alcohol, 64,* 607–615.

Karno, M. P., & Longabaugh, R. (2004). What do we know? Process analysis and the search for a better understanding of Project MATCH's Anger-by-Treatment matching effect. *Journal of Studies on Alcohol, 65,* 501–512.

Karno, M. P., & Longabaugh, R. (2005a). An examination of how therapist directiveness interacts with patient anger and reactance to predict alcohol use. *Journal of Studies on Alcohol, 66,* 825–832.

Karno, M. P., & Longabaugh, R. (2005b). Less directiveness by therapists improves drinking outcomes of reactant clients in alcoholism treatment. *Journal of Consulting and Clinical Psychology, 73,* 262–267.

Kazdin, A. E., & Nock, M. K. (2003). Delineating mechanisms of change in child and adolescent therapy: Methodological issues and research recommendations. *Journal of Child Psychology and Psychiatry, 44,* 1116–29.

Kidorf, M., Neufeld, K., & Brooner, R. K. (2004). Combining stepped care approaches with behavioral reinforcement to motivate employment in opioid-dependent outpatients. *Substance Use and Misuse, 39,* 2215–2238

King, V. L., Stoller, K. B., Hayes, M., Umbricht, A., Currens, M., Kidorf, M., et al. (2002). A multicenter randomized evaluation of methadone medical maintenance. *Drug and Alcohol Dependence, 65,* 137–148.

Kissin, W., McLeod, C., & McKay, J. R. (2003). The longitudinal relationship between self-help attendance and course of recovery. *Evaluation and Program Planning, 25,* 311–324.

Koenig, L., Siegel, J. M., Harwood, H., Gilani, J., Chen, Y., Leahy, P., et al. (2005). Economic benefits of substance abuse treatment: Findings from Cuyahoga County, Ohio. *Journal of Substance Abuse Treatment, 28*(Suppl. 1), S41-S50.

Koob, G. F. (2000). Stress, corticotropin-releasing factor and drug addiction. *Annals of the New York Academy of Science, 897*(Suppl. 1), 27–45.

Koob, G. F. (2003). Neuroadaptive mechanisms of addiction: Studies on the extended amygdala. *European Neuropsychopharmacology, 13*, 442–452.

Koob, G. F. (2006). The neurobiology of addiction: A neuroadaptational view relevant for diagnosis. *Addiction, 101*(Suppl. 1), 23–30.

Krahn, M., & Naglie, G. (2008). The next step in guideline development: Incorporating patient preferences. *JAMA, 200*, 436–438.

Kranzler, H. R., Armeli, S., Feinn, R., & Tennen, H. (2004). Targeted naltrexone treatment moderates the relations between mood and drinking behavior among problem drinkers. *Journal of Consulting and Clinical Psychology, 72,* 317–327.

Kranzler, H. R., Armeli, S., Tennen, H., Blomqvist, O., Oncken, C., Petry, N., et al. (2003). Targeted naltrexone for early problem drinkers. *Journal of Clinical Psychopharmacology, 23*, 294–304.

Kreek, M. J., Nielsen, D. A., Butelman, E. R., & LaForge, K. S. (2005). Genetic influences on impulsivity, risk taking, stress responsivity and vulnerability to drug abuse and addiction. *Nature Neuroscience, 8*, 1450–1457.

Kristenson, H., Ohlin, H., Hulten-Nosslin, M. B., Trell, E., & Hood, B. (1983). Identification and intervention of heavy drinking in middle-aged men: Results and follow-up of 24–60 months of long-term study with randomized controls. *Alcoholism: Clinical and Experimental Research, 7*, 203–209.

Kristenson, H., Osterling, A., Nilsson, J. A., & Lindgarde, F. (2002). Prevention of alcohol-related deaths in middle-aged heavy drinkers. *Alcoholism: Clinical and Experimental Research, 26*, 478–484.

Krystal, J. H., Cramer, J. A., Krol, W. F., & Kirk, G. F. (2001). Naltrexone in the treatment of alcohol dependence. *New England Journal of Medicine, 345*, 1734–1739.

Lambert, M. J., Hansen, N. B. & Finch, A. E. (2001). Patient-focused research: Using patient outcome data to enhance treatment effects. *Journal of Consulting and Clinical Psychology, 69*, 159–172.

Lambert, M. J., Whipple, J. L., Smart, D. W., Vermeersch, D. A., Nielsen, S. L., & Hawkins, E. J. (2001). The effects of providing therapists with feedback on patient progress during psychotherapy: Are outcomes enhanced? *Psychotherapy Research, 11*, 49–68.

Lash, S. J. (1998). Increasing participation in substance abuse aftercare treatment. *American Journal of Drug and Alcohol Abuse, 24*, 31–36.

Lash, S. J., & Blosser, S. L. (1999). Increasing adherence to substance abuse aftercare group therapy. *Journal of Substance Abuse Treatment, 16*, 55–60.

Lash, S. J., Burden, J. L., & Fearer, S. A. (2007). Contracting, prompting, and reinforcing substance abuse treatment aftercare adherence. *Journal of Drug Addiction, Education, and Eradication, 2*, 455–490.

Lash, S. J., Burden, J. L., Monteleone, B. R., & Lehmann, L. P. (2004). Social reinforcement of substance abuse treatment aftercare participation: Impact on outcome. *Addictive Behaviors, 29*, 337–342.

Lash, S. J., Petersen, G. E., O'Connor, E. A., & Lehmann, L. P. (2001). Social reinforcement of substance abuse aftercare group therapy attendance. *Journal of Substance Abuse Treatment, 20*, 3–8.

Lash, S. J., Stephens, R. S., Burden, J. L., Grambow, S. C., DeMarce, J. M., Jones, M. E., et al. (2007). Contracting, prompting, and reinforcing substance use disorder continuing care: A randomized clinical trial. *Psychology of Addictive Behaviors, 21*, 387–397.

Lavori, P. W., & Dawson, R. (2004). Dynamic treatment regimes: Practical design considerations. *Clinical Trials, 1*, 9–20.

Lavori, P. W., Dawson, R., & Rush, A. J. (2000). Flexible treatment strategies in chronic disease: Clinical and research implications. *Biological Psychiatry, 48*, 605–614.

Li, C. S., & Sinha, R. (2008). Inhibitory control and emotional stress regulation: Neuroimaging evidence for frontal-limbic dysfunction in psycho-stimulant addiction. *Neuroscience and Biobehavioral Reviews, 32*, 581–597.

Lieber, C. S., Weiss, D. G., Groszmann, R., Paronetto, F., & Schenker, S. (2003). Veterans Affairs Cooperative Study of Polyenylphosphatidylcholine in Alcoholic Liver Disease: Effects on drinking behavior by nurse/physician teams. *Alcoholism: Clinical and Experimental Research, 27*, 1757–1764.

Litt, M. D., Kadden, R. M., Cooney, N., & Kabela, E. (2003). Coping skills and treatment outcomes in cognitive–behavioral and interactional group therapy for alcoholism. *Journal of Consulting and Clinical Psychology, 71*, 118–128.

Litt, M. D., Kadden, R. M., Kabela-Cormier, E., & Petry, N. (2007). Changing network support for drinking: Initial findings from the network support project. *Journal of Consulting and Clinical Psychology, 75*, 542–555.

Longabaugh, R., & Morgenstern, J. (1999). Cognitive–behavioral coping-skills therapy for alcohol dependence: Current status and future directions. *Alcohol Research and Health, 23*, 78–85.

Longabaugh, R., & Wirtz, P. W. (2001). Substantive review and critique. In R. Longabaugh & P. W. Wirtz (Eds.), *Project MATCH hypotheses: Results and causal chain analyses* (pp. 305–325). Bethesda, MD: U.S. Department of Health and Human Services.

Longabaugh, R., Wirtz, P. W., Beattie, M. C., Noel, N., & Stout, R. L. (1995). Matching treatment focus to patient social investment and support: 18-month follow-up results. *Journal of Consulting and Clinical Psychology, 63*, 296–307.

Longabaugh, R., Wirtz, P. W., & Connors, G. (2001). Network support for drinking. In R. Longabaugh & P. W. Wirtz (Eds.), *Project MATCH hypotheses: Results and causal chain analyses* (pp. 260–275). Bethesda, MD: U.S. Department of Health and Human Services.

Lueger, R. J., Howard, K. I., Martinovich, Z., Lutz, W., Anderson, E. E., & Grissom, G. (2001). Assessing treatment progress of individual patients using expected treatment response models. *Journal of Consulting and Clinical Psychology, 69*, 150–158.

Lussier, J. P., Heil, S. H., Mongeon, J. A., Badger, G. J., & Higgins, S. T. (2006). A meta-analysis of voucher-based reinforcement therapy for substance use disorders. *Addiction, 101*, 192–203.

Lynch, K. G., Courtright, L., Zaharakis, N., Kampman, K., Pettinati, H. M., McKay, J. R., et al. (2009, June). *Extending treatment effectiveness of naltrexone: A sequential randomized trial.* Poster presented at the Research Society on Alcoholism conference, San Diego, CA.

MacKinnon, D. P., Lockwood, C. M., Hoffman, J. M., West, S. G., & Sheets, U. (2002). A comparison of methods to test mediation and other intervening variable effects. *Psychological Methods, 7*, 83–104.

Magura, S., Staines, G., Kosanke, N., Rosenblum, A., Foote, J., Deluca, A., et al. (2003). Predictive validity of the ASAM patient placement criteria for naturalistically matched vs. mismatched alcoholism patients. *American Journal on Addictions, 12*, 386–397.

Marijuana Treatment Project Research Group. (2004). Brief treatments for cannabis dependence: Findings from a randomized multisite trial. *Journal of Consulting and Clinical Psychology, 72*, 455–466.

Marlatt, G. A., & Gordon, J. R. (1985). *Relapse prevention: Maintenance strategies in the treatment of addictive behaviors.* New York: Guilford Press.

Marlowe, D. B., Festinger, D. S., Arabia, P. L., Dugosh, K. L., Benasutti, K. M., Croft, J. R., et al. (2008). Adaptive interventions in drug court: A pilot experiment. *Criminal Justice Review, 33*, 343–360.

Marlowe, D. B., Festinger, D. S., Dugosh, K. L., Lee, P. A., & Benasutti, K. M. (2007). Adapting judicial supervision to the risk level of drug offenders: Discharge and 6-month outcomes from a prospective matching study. *Drug and Alcohol Dependence, 88*(Suppl. 2), S4–S13.

Marlowe, D. B., Festinger, D. S., Lee, P. A., Schepise, M. M., Hazzard, J. E. R., Merrill, J. C., et al. (2003). Are judicial status hearings a key component of drug court? During-treatment data from a randomized trial. *Criminal Justice and Behavior, 30*, 141–162.

Martell, B. A., Mitchell, E., Poling, J., Gonsai, K., & Kosten, T. R. (2005). Vaccine pharmacotherapy for the treatment of cocaine dependence. *Biological Psychiatry, 58*, 158–164.

Mattson, M. E., Allen, J. P., Longabaugh, R., Nickless, C. J., Connors, G. J., & Kadden, R. M. (1994). A chronological review of empirical studies matching alcoholic clients to treatment. *Journal of Studies on Alcohol, 12*, 16–29.

Maude-Griffin, P., Hohenstein, J., Humfleet, G., Reilly, P., Tusel, D., & Hall, S. (1998). Superior efficacy of cognitive–behavioral therapy for urban crack cocaine abusers: Main and matching effects. *Journal of Consulting and Clinical Psychology, 66*, 832–837.

McAuliffe, W. E. (1990). A randomized controlled trial of recovery training and self-help for opioid addicts in New England and Hong Kong. *Journal of Psychoactive Drugs, 22*, 197–209.

McAuliffe, W. E., & Ch'ien, J. M. N. (1986). Recovery training and self-help: A relapse prevention program for treated opiate addicts. *Journal of Substance Abuse Treatment, 3*, 9–20.

McElrath, D. (1997). The Minnesota model. *Journal of Psychoactive Drugs, 29*, 141–144.

McKay, J. R. (1999). Studies of factors in relapse to alcohol and drug use: A critical review of methodologies and findings. *Journal of Studies on Alcohol, 60*, 566–576.

McKay, J. R. (2001a). Effectiveness of continuing care interventions for substance abusers: Implications for the study of long-term treatment effects. *Evaluation Review, 25*, 211–232.

McKay, J. R. (2001b). The role of continuing care in outpatient alcohol treatment programs. In M. Galanter (Ed.), *Recent developments in alcoholism: Vol. 15. Services research in the era of managed care* (pp. 357–372). New York: Kluwer Academic/Plenum Press.

McKay, J. R. (2005). Is there a case for extended interventions for alcohol and drug use disorders? *Addiction, 100*, 1594–1610.

McKay, J. R. (2006). Continuing care in the treatment of addictive disorders. *Current Psychiatry Reports, 8*, 355–362.

McKay, J. R. (2007). Lessons learned from psychotherapy research. *Alcoholism: Clinical and Experimental Research, 31*(Suppl. 3), 48–54.

McKay, J. R. (2009). Continuing care research: What we have learned and where we are going. *Journal of Substance Abuse Treatment, 36*, 131–145.

McKay, J. R., Alterman, A. I., Cacciola, J. S., Mulvaney, F. D., & O'Brien, C. P. (2000). Prognostic significance of antisocial personality in cocaine-dependent patients entering continuing care. *Journal of Nervous and Mental Disease, 188*, 287–296.

McKay, J. R., Alterman, A. I., Cacciola, J. S., O'Brien, C. P., Koppenhaver, J. M., & Shepard, D. S. (1999). Continuing care for cocaine dependence: Comprehensive 2-year outcomes. *Journal of Consulting and Clinical Psychology, 67*, 420–427.

McKay, J. R., Alterman, A. I., Cacciola, J. S., Rutherford, M., O'Brien, C. P., & Koppenhaver, J. M. (1997). Group counseling versus individualized relapse prevention aftercare following intensive outpatient treatment for cocaine dependence: Initial results. *Journal of Consulting and Clinical Psychology, 65*, 778–788.

McKay, J. R., Alterman, A. I., Koppenhaver, J., Mulvaney, F., Bovasso, G., & Ward, K. (2001). Continuous, categorical, and time to event cocaine use outcome variables: Degree of intercorrelation and sensitivity to treatment group differences. *Drug and Alcohol Dependence, 62*, 19–30.

McKay, J. R., Alterman, A. I., McLellan, A. T., Boardman, C., Mulvaney, F., & O'Brien, C. P. (1998). The effect of random versus non-random assignment in the evaluation of treatment for cocaine abusers. *Journal of Consulting and Clinical Psychology, 66*, 697–701.

McKay, J. R., Cacciola, J., McLellan, A. T., Alterman, A. I., & Wirtz, P. W. (1997). An initial evaluation of the psychosocial dimensions of the ASAM criteria for inpatient and day hospital substance abuse rehabilitation. *Journal of Studies on Alcohol, 58,* 239–252.

McKay, J. R., Carise, D., Dennis, M. L., Dupont, R., Humphreys, K., Kemp, J., et al. (2009). Extending the benefits of addiction treatment: Practical strategies for continuing care and recovery. *Journal of Substance Abuse Treatment, 36,* 127–130.

McKay, J. R., Foltz, C., Leahy, P., Stephens, R., Orwin, R., & Crowley, E. (2004). Step down continuing care in the treatment of substance abuse: Correlates of participation and outcome effects. *Evaluation and Program Planning, 27,* 321–331.

McKay, J. R., Franklin, T. R., Patapis, N., & Lynch, K. G. (2006). Conceptual, methodological, and analytical issues in the study of relapse. *Clinical Psychology Review, 26,* 109–127.

McKay, J. R., Long, M., Lynch, K., Van Horn, D., & Oslin, D. (2008, October). *Effectiveness of extended telephone continuing care.* Paper presented at the Association of Health Services Research, Boston, MA.

McKay, J. R., Lynch, K. G., Coviello, D., Morrison, R., & Dackis, C. (2008, June). *Effectiveness of contingency management and CBT in intensive outpatient treatment for cocaine dependence.* Poster presented at the College on Problems of Drug Dependence, San Juan, Puerto Rico.

McKay, J. R., Lynch, K. G., Morrison, R., & Coviello, D. (2009). *Challenges in implementing contingency management and extra services matched to problems in intensive outpatient treatment for cocaine dependence.* Manuscript in preparation, University of Pennsylvania.

McKay, J. R., Lynch, K. G., Shepard, D. S., Morgenstern, J., Forman, R. F., & Pettinati, H. M. (2005). Do patient characteristics and initial progress in treatment moderate the effectiveness of telephone-based continuing care for substance use disorders? *Addiction, 100,* 216–226.

McKay, J. R., Lynch, K. G., Shepard, D. S., & Pettinati, H. M. (2005). The effectiveness of telephone-based continuing care for alcohol and cocaine dependence: 24-month outcomes. *Archives of General Psychiatry, 62,* 199–207.

McKay, J. R., Lynch, K. G., Shepard, D. S., Ratichek, S., Morrison, R., Koppenhaver, J., & Pettinati, H. M. (2004). The effectiveness of telephone-based continuing care in the clinical management of alcohol and cocaine use disorders: 12-month outcomes. *Journal of Consulting and Clinical Psychology, 72,* 967–979.

McKay, J. R., Lynch, K. G., Van Horn, D., Ivey, M., Oslin, D. W., & Drapkin, M. (2009, June). *Effectiveness of extended telephone continuing care: 18-month outcomes.* Poster presented at the Research Society on Alcoholism conference, San Diego, CA.

McKay, J. R., Lynch, K. G., Van Horn, D., Ward, K., & Oslin, D. (2008, June–July). *Effectiveness of extended telephone continuing care.* Poster presented at the Research Society on Alcoholism conference, Washington, DC.

McKay, J. R., Merikle, E., Mulvaney, F. D., Weiss, R. V., & Koppenhaver, J. M. (2001). Factors accounting for cocaine use two years following initiation of continuing care. *Addiction, 96,* 213–225.

McKay, J. R., & Weiss, R. V. (2001). A review of temporal effects and outcome predictors in substance abuse treatment studies with long-term follow-ups: Preliminary results and methodological issues. *Evaluation Review, 25,* 113–161.

McKinnon, D. P., & Lockwood, C. M. (2003). Advances in statistical methods for substance abuse prevention research. *Prevention Science, 4,* 155–171.

McLatchie, B. H., & Lomp, K. G. E. (1988). An experimental investigation of the influence of aftercare on alcoholic relapse. *British Journal of Addiction, 83,* 1045–1054.

McLellan, A. T., Arndt, I. O., Metzger, D. S., Woody, G. E, & O'Brien, C. P. (1993). The effects of psychosocial services in substance abuse treatment. *JAMA, 269,* 1953–1959.

McLellan, A. T., Carise, D., & Kleber, H. D. (2003). The national addiction treatment infrastructure: Can it support the public's demand for quality care? *Journal of Substance Abuse Treatment, 25,* 117–121.

McLellan, A. T., Grissom, G. R., Zanis, D., Randall, M., Brill, P., & O'Brien, C. P. (1997). Problem-service "matching" in addiction treatment: A prospective study in 4 programs. *Archives of General Psychiatry, 54,* 730–735.

McLellan, A. T., Hagan, T. A., Levine, M., Gould, F., Meyers, K., Bencivengo, M., et al. (1998). Supplemental social services improve outcomes in public addiction treatment. *Addiction, 93,* 1489–1499.

McLellan, A. T., Kemp, J., Brooks, A., & Carise, D. (2008). Improving public addiction treatment through performance contracting: The Delaware experiment. *Health Policy, 87,* 296–308.

McLellan, A. T., Lewis, D. C., O'Brien, C. P., & Kleber, H. D. (2000). Drug dependence, a chronic medical illness: Implications for treatment, insurance, and outcomes evaluation. *JAMA, 284,* 1689–1695.

McLellan, A. T., Luborsky, L., Woody, G. E., O'Brien, C. P., & Druley, K. A. (1983). Predicting response to alcohol and drug abuse treatments: Role of psychiatric severity. *Archives of General Psychiatry, 40,* 620–625.

McLellan, A. T., McKay, J. R., Forman, R., Cacciola, J., & Kemp, J. (2005). Reconsidering the evaluation of addiction treatment: From retrospective follow-up to concurrent recovery monitoring. *Addiction, 100,* 447–458.

McLellan, A. T., & Meyers, K. (2004). Contemporary addiction treatment: A review of systems problems for adults and adolescents. *Biological Psychiatry, 56,* 764–770.

McLellan, A. T., Skipper, G. S., Campbell, M., & DuPont, R. L. (2008, November 4). Five-year outcomes in a cohort study of physicians treated for substance use disorders in the United States. *BMJ, 337,* a2038.

Mensinger, J. L., Lynch, K. G., Ten Have, T. R., & McKay, J. R. (2007). Mediators of telephone-based continuing care for alcohol and cocaine dependence. *Journal of Consulting and Clinical Psychology, 75,* 775–784.

Metzger, D. S., Platt, J. J., Zanis, D., & Fureman, I. (1992). *Vocational problem solving: A structured intervention for unemployed substance abuse treatment clients.* Philadelphia: University of Pennsylvania/Hahnemann University School of Medicine.

Meyers, R. J., & Smith, J. E. (1995). *Clinical guide to alcohol treatment: The community reinforcement approach.* New York: Guilford Press.

Milby, J. B., Schumacher, J. E., McNamara, C., Wallace, D., Usdan, S., McGill, T., & Michael, M. (2000). Initiating abstinence in cocaine abusing dually diagnosed homeless persons. *Drug and Alcohol Dependence, 60*, 55–67.

Milby, J. B., Schumacher, J. E., Raczynski, J. M., Caldwell, E., Engle, M., Michael, M., & Carr, J. (1996). Sufficient conditions for effective treatment of substance abusing homeless persons. *Drug and Alcohol Dependence, 43*, 39–47.

Milby, J. B., Schumacher, J. E., Wallace, D., Freedman, M. J., & Vuchinich, R. E. (2005). To house or not to house: The effects of providing housing to homeless substance abusers in treatment. *American Journal of Public Health, 95*, 1259–1265.

Milby, J. B., Schumacher, J. E., Wallace, D., Frison, J., McNamara, C., Usdan, S., & Michael, M. (2003). Day treatment with contingency management for cocaine abuse in homeless persons: 12-month follow-up. *Journal of Consulting and Clinical Psychology, 71*, 619–621.

Miller, W. R., & Manuel, J. K. (2008). How large must a treatment effect be before it matters to practitioners? An estimation method and demonstration. *Drug and Alcohol Review, 27*, 524–528.

Miller, W. R., & Rollnick, S. (2002). *Motivational interviewing: Preparing people for change* (2nd ed.). New York: Guilford Press.

Miller, W. R., & Weisner, C. (2002). Integrated care. In W. R. Miller & C. M. Weisner (Eds.), *Changing substance abuse through health and social systems* (pp. 243–253). New York: Kluwer Academic/Plenum Press.

Miller, W. R., Westerberg, V. S., Harris, R. J., & Tonigan, J. S. (1996). What predicts relapse? Prospective testing of antecedent models. *Addiction, 91*(Suppl. 12), S155–S172.

Miller, W. R., & Wilbourne, P. L. (2002). Mesa Grande: A methodological analysis of clinical trials of treatments for alcohol use disorders. *Addiction, 97*, 265–277.

Miller, W. R., Yahne, C. E., & Tonigan, J. S. (2003). Motivational interviewing in drug abuse services: A randomized trial. *Journal of Consulting and Clinical Psychology, 71*, 754–763.

Monti, P. M., Abrams, D. B., Kadden, R. M., & Cooney, N. L. (1989). *Treating alcohol dependence: A coping skills training guide.* New York: Guilford Press.

Monti, P. M., Colby, S. M., Barnett, N. P., Spirito, A., Rohsenow, D. J., Myers, M., et al. (1999). Brief intervention for harm reduction with alcohol-positive older adolescents in a hospital emergency department. *Journal of Consulting and Clinical Psychology, 67*, 989–994.

Monti, P. M., Miranda, R., Jr., Nixon, K., Sher, K. J., Swartzwelder, H. S., Tapert, S. F., et al. (2005). Adolescence: Booze, brains, and behavior. *Alcoholism: Clinical and Experimental Research, 29*, 207–220.

Moos, R. H., Finney, J. W., & Cronkite, R. C. (1990). *Alcoholism treatment: Context, process, and outcome.* New York: Oxford University Press.

Moos, R. H., & Moos, B. S. (2004). Long-term influence of duration and frequency of participation in Alcoholics Anonymous on individuals with alcohol use disorders. *Journal of Consulting and Clinical Psychology, 72,* 81–90.

Moos, R. H., & Moos, B. S. (2007). Treated and untreated alcohol-use disorders: Course and predictors of remission and relapse. *Evaluation Review: A Journal of Applied Social Research, 31,* 564–584.

Morgenstern, J., Blanchard, K. A., McCrady, B. S., McVeigh, K. H., Morgan, T. J., & Pandina, R. J. (2006). Effectiveness of intensive case management for substance-dependent women receiving temporary assistance for needy families. *American Journal of Public Health, 96,* 2016–2023.

Morgenstern, J., Bux, D., Labouvie, E., Morgan, T. J., Blanchard, K. A., & Muench, F. (2003). Examining mechanisms of action in 12-step community outpatient treatment. *Drug and Alcohol Dependence, 72,* 237–247.

Morgenstern, J., Hogue, A., Dauber, S., Dasaro, C., & McKay, J. R. (in press). A practical clinical trial of care management to treat substance use disorders among public assistance beneficiaries. *Journal of Consulting and Clinical Psychology.*

Morgenstern, J., Labouvie, E., McCrady, B., Kahler, C., & Frey, R. (1997). Affiliation with Alcoholics Anonymous following treatment: A study of its therapeutic effects and mechanisms of action. *Journal of Consulting and Clinical Psychology, 65,* 768–778.

Morgenstern, J., & Longabaugh, R. (2000). Cognitive–behavioral treatment for alcohol dependence: A review of evidence for its hypothesized mechanisms of action. *Addiction, 95,* 1475–1490.

Morgenstern, J., & McKay, J. R. (2007). Rethinking the paradigms that inform behavioral treatment research for substance use disorders. *Addiction, 102,* 1377–1389.

Moyers, T. B., Miller, W. R., & Hendrickson, S. M. (2005). How does motivational interviewing work? Therapist interpersonal skill predicts client involvement within motivational interviewing sessions. *Journal of Consulting and Clinical Psychology, 73,* 590–598.

Murphy, S. A. (2003). Optimal dynamic treatment regimes. *Journal of the Royal Statistical Society: Series B, 65,* 331–366.

Murphy, S. A. (2005). An experimental design for the development of adaptive treatment strategies. *Statistics in Medicine, 24,* 1455–1481.

Murphy, S. A., Lynch, K. G., McKay, J. R., Oslin, D. W., & Ten Have, T. R. (2007). Developing adaptive treatment strategies in substance abuse research. *Drug and Alcohol Dependence, 88*(Suppl. 2), S24–S30.

Murphy, S. A., & McKay, J. R. (2004, Winter/Spring). Adaptive treatment strategies: An emerging approach for improving treatment effectiveness. *Clinical Science,* 7–13.

Nestler, E. J. (2005). Is there a common molecular pathway for addiction? *Nature Neuroscience, 8,* 1445–1449.

Nierenberg, A. A., Fava, M., Trivedi, M. H., Wisniewski, S. R., Thase, M. E., McGrath, P. M., et al. (2006). A comparison of lithium and T(3) augmentation following two failed medication treatments for depression: A STAR*D report. *The American Journal of Psychiatry, 163*, 1519–1530.

Nowinski, J., Baker, S., & Carroll, K. M. (1995). *Twelve step facilitation therapy manual* (NIH Publication No. 94-3722). Rockville, MD: National Institute on Alcohol Abuse and Alcoholism.

Obernier, J. A., White, A. M., Swartzwelder, H. S., & Crews, F. T. (2002). Cognitive deficits and CNS damage after a 4-day binge ethanol exposure in rats. *Pharmacology, Biochemistry, and Behavior, 72*, 521–532.

O'Brien, C. P., & McKay, J. R. (2007). Psychopharmacological treatments of substance use disorders. In P. E. Nathan & J. M. Gorman (Eds.), *A guide to treatments that work* (3rd ed., pp. 145–178). New York: Oxford University Press.

O'Farrell, T. J., Choquette, K. A., & Cutter, H. S. G. (1998). Couples relapse prevention sessions after behavioral marital therapy for male alcoholics: Outcomes during the three years after starting treatment. *Journal of Studies on Alcohol, 59*, 357–370.

O'Farrell, T. J., & Fals-Stewart, W. (2001). Family-involved alcoholism treatment: An update. In M. Galanter (Ed.), *Recent developments in alcoholism: Volume 15. Services research in the era of managed care* (pp. 329–356). New York: Kluwer Academic/Plenum Press.

Office of National Drug Control Policy. (2004). *The economic costs of drug abuse in the United States, 1992–2002* (Publication No. 207303). Washington, DC: Executive Office of the President.

O'Malley, S. S., Garbutt, J. C., Gastfriend, D. R., Dong, Q., & Kranzler, H. R. (2007). Efficacy of extended-release naltrexone in alcohol-dependent patients who are abstinent before treatment. *Journal of Clinical Psychopharmacology, 27*, 507–512.

O'Malley, S. S., Rounsaville, B. J., Farren, C., Namkoong, K., Wu, R., Robinson, J., et al. (2003). Initial and maintenance naltrexone treatment for alcohol dependence using primary care vs. specialty care. *Archives of Internal Medicine, 163*, 1695–1704.

Orford, J., Hodgson, R., Copello, A., John, B., Smith, M., Black, R., et al., (2006). The clients' perspective on change during treatment for an alcohol problem: Qualitative analysis of follow-up interviews in the UK Alcohol Treatment Trial. *Addiction, 101*, 60–68.

Orlinsky, D. E., Ronnestad, M. H., & Willutzki, U. (2004). Fifty years of psychotherapy process-outcome research: Continuity and change. In M. Lambert (Ed.), *Handbook of psychotherapy and behavior change* (5th ed., pp. 307–391). New York: Wiley.

Oslin, D. W., Berrettini, W., Kranzler, H. R., Pettinati, H., Gelernter, J., Volpicelli, J. R., & O'Brien, C. P. (2003). A functional polymorphism of the μ-opioid receptor gene is associated with naltrexone response in alcohol-dependent patients. *Neuropsychopharmacology, 28*, 1546–1552.

Oslin, D. W., Ross, J., Sayers, S., Murphy, J., Kane, V., & Katz, I. R. (2006). Screening, assessment, and management of depression in VA primary care clinics. *Journal of General Internal Medicine, 21*, 46–50.

Otto, M. W., Pollack, M. H., & Maki, K. M. (2000). Empirically supported treatments for panic disorder: Costs, benefits, and stepped care. *Journal of Consulting and Clinical Psychology, 68*, 556–563.

Ouimette, P. C., Moos, R. H., & Finney, J. W. (1998). Influence of outpatient treatment and 12-step group involvement on one-year substance abuse treatment outcome. *Journal of Studies on Alcohol, 59*, 513–522.

Patterson, D. G., MacPherson, J., & Brady, N. M. (1997). Community psychiatric nurse aftercare for alcoholics: A five-year follow-up study. *Addiction, 92*, 459–468.

Petry, N. M. (2000). A comprehensive guide to the application of contingency management procedures in clinical settings. *Drug and Alcohol Dependence, 58*, 9–26.

Petry, N. M., Alessi, S. M., & Hanson, T. (2007). Contingency management improves abstinence and quality of life in cocaine abusers. *Journal of Consulting and Clinical Psychology, 75*, 307–315.

Pettinati, H. M., Weiss, R. D., Miller, W. R., Donovan, D., Ernst, D. B., & Rounsaville, B. J. (2004). *Medical management (MM) treatment manual*. Bethesda, MD: National Institute on Alcohol Abuse and Alcoholism.

Pfefferbaum, A., Sullivan, E. V., Mathalon, D. H., Shear, P. K., Rosenbloom, M. J., & Lim, K. O. (1995). Longitudinal changes in magnetic resonance imaging brain volumes in abstinent and relapsed alcoholics. *Alcoholism: Clinical and Experimental Research, 19*, 1177–1191.

Popovici, I., French, M. T., & McKay, J. R. (2008). Economic evaluation of continuing care interventions in the treatment of substance abuse: Recommendations for future research. *Evaluation Review, 32*, 547–568.

Prendergast, M., Podus, D., Finney, J., Greenwell, L., & Roll, J. (2006). Contingency management for treatment of substance use disorders: A meta-analysis. *Addiction, 101*, 1546–1650.

Project MATCH Research Group. (1997). Matching alcoholism treatments to client heterogeneity: Project MATCH posttreatment drinking outcomes. *Journal of Studies on Alcoholism, 58*, 7–29.

Rakowski, W., Lipkus, I. M., Clark, M. A., Rimer, B. K., Ehrich, B., Lyna, P. R., et al. (2003). Reminder letter, tailored stepped-care, and self-choice comparison for repeat mammography. *American Journal of Preventive Medicine, 25*, 308–314.

Rapp, R. C., Xu, J., Carr, C. A., Lane, D. T., Wang, J., & Carlson, R. (2006). Treatment barriers identified by substance abusers assessed at a centralized intake unit. *Journal of Substance Abuse Treatment, 30*, 227–235.

Rawson, R. A., Marinelli-Casey, P., Anglin, M. D., Dickow, A., Frazier, Y., Gallagher, C., et al. (2004). A multi-site comparison of psychosocial approaches for the treatment of methamphetamine dependence. *Addiction, 99*, 708–717.

Rawson, R. A., Shoptaw, S. J., Obert, J. L., McCann, M. J., Hasson, A. L., Marinelli-Casey, P. J., et al. (1995). An intensive outpatient approach for cocaine abuse treatment. *Journal of Substance Abuse Treatment, 12*, 117–127.

Rhodes, G. L., Saules, K. K., Helmus, T. C., Roll, J. M., BeShears, R. S., Ledgerwood, D. M., et al. (2003). Improving on-time counseling attendance in a methadone treatment program: A contingency management approach. *American Journal of Drug and Alcohol Abuse, 29,* 759–773.

Rohsenow, D., Monti, P., Martin, R., Michalec, E., & Abrams, D. (2000). Brief coping skills treatment for cocaine abuse: 12-month substance use outcomes. *Journal of Consulting and Clinical Psychology, 68,* 515–520.

Rosenman, M. B., Holmes, A. M., Ackermann, R. T., Murray, M. D., Doebbeling, C. C., Katz, B., et al. (2006). The Indiana chronic disease management program. *Milbank Quarterly, 84,* 135–163.

Rothman, A. J. (2000). Toward a theory-based analysis of behavioral maintenance. *Health Psychology, 19*(Suppl.), 64–69.

Rush, A. J., Fava, M., Wisniewski, S. R., Lavori, P. W., Trivedi, M. H., Sackeim, H. A., et al. (2004). Sequenced treatment alternatives to relieve depression (STAR*D): Rational and design. *Controlled Clinical Trials, 25,* 119–142.

Rush, A. J., Trivedi, M. H., Wisniewski, S. R., Stewart, J. W., Nierenberg, A. A., Thase, M. E., et al. (2006). Buproprion-SR, sertraline, or venlafaxine-XR after failure of SSRIs for depression. *New England Journal of Medicine, 354,* 1231–1242.

Saitz, R., Horton, N. J., Larson, M. J., Winter, M., & Samet, J. H. (2005). Primary medical care and reductions in addiction severity: A prospective cohort study. *Addiction, 100,* 70–78.

Samet, J. H., Larson, M. J., Horton, N. J., Doyle, K., Winter, M., & Saitz, R. (2003). Linking alcohol- and drug-dependent adults to primary medical care: A randomized controlled trial of a multi-disciplinary health intervention in a detoxification unit. *Addiction, 98,* 509–516.

Sannibale, C., Hurkett, P., Van Den Bossche, E., O'Connor, D., Zador, D., Capus, C., et al. (2003). Aftercare attendance and post-treatment functioning of severely substance dependent residential treatment clients. *Drug and Alcohol Review, 22,* 181–190.

Saxon, A. J., Malte, C. A., Sloan, K. L., Baer, J. S., Calsyn, D. A., Nichol, P., et al. (2006). Randomized trial of onsite versus referral primary medical care for veterans in addictions treatment. *Medical Care, 44,* 334–342.

Schaefer, J. A., Ingudomnukul, E., Harris, A. H. S., & Cronkite, R. C. (2005). Continuity of care practices and substance use disorder patients' engagement in continuing care. *Medical Care, 43,* 1234–1241.

Schmitt, S. K., Phibbs, C. S., & Piette, J. D. (2003). The influence of distance on utilization of outpatient mental health aftercare following inpatient substance abuse treatment. *Addictive Behaviors, 28,* 1183–1192.

Schmitz, J. M., Oswald, L. M., Jacks, S. D., Rustin, T., Rhoades, H. M., & Grabowski, J. (1997). Relapse prevention treatment for cocaine dependence: Group vs. individual format. *Addictive Behaviors, 22,* 405–418.

Scogin, F. R., Hanson, A., & Welsh, D. (2003). Self-administered treatment in stepped-care models of depression treatment. *Journal of Clinical Psychology, 59,* 341–349.

Scott, C. K. (2004). A replicable model for achieving over 90% follow-up rates in longitudinal studies of substance abusers. *Drug and Alcohol Dependence, 74*, 21–36.

Scott, C. K., & Dennis, M. L. (2002). *Recovery Management Checkup (RMC) protocol for people with chronic substance use disorders.* Bloomington, IL: Chestnut Health Systems.

Scott, C. K., & Dennis, M. L. (in press). Results from two randomized clinical trials evaluating the impact of quarterly recovery management checkups with adult chronic substance users. *Addiction.*

Scott, C. K., Dennis, M. L., & Foss, M. A. (2005). Utilizing recovery management checkups to shorten the cycle of relapse, treatment reentry, and recovery. *Drug and Alcohol Dependence, 78*, 325–338.

Sees, K. L., Delucchi, K. L., Masson, C., Rosen, A., Clark, H. W., Robillard, H., et al. (2000). Methadone maintenance vs. 180-day psychosocially enriched detoxification for treatment of opioid dependence: A randomized controlled trial. *JAMA, 283*, 1303–1310.

Shaham, Y., & Hope, B. T. (2005). The role of neuroadaptations in relapse to drug seeking. *Nature Neuroscience, 8*, 1437–1439.

Shadish, W. R., & Baldwin, S. A. (2005). Effects of behavioral marital therapy: A meta-analysis of randomized controlled trials. *Journal of Consulting and Clinical Psychology, 73*, 6–14.

Shepard, D. S., Calabro, J. A. B., Love, C. T., McKay, J. R., Tetreault, J., & Yeom, H. S. (2006). Counselor incentives to improve client retention in an outpatient substance abuse aftercare program. *Administration and Policy in Mental Health & Mental Health Services Research, 33*, 629–635.

Shiffman, S., Balabanis, M. H., Paty, J. A., Engberg, J., Gwaltney, C. J., Liu, K. S., et al. (2000). Dynamic effects of self-efficacy on smoking lapse and relapse. *Health Psychology, 19*, 315–323.

Shiffman, S., Hickcox, M., Paty, J. A., Gnys, M., Kassel J. D., & Richards, T. J. (1996). Progression from a smoking lapse to relapse: Prediction from abstinence violation effects, nicotine dependence, and lapse characteristics. *Journal of Consulting and Clinical Psychology, 64*, 993–1002.

Shiffman, S., Hufford, M., Hickcox, M., Paty, J. A., Gnys, M., & Kassel, J. D. (1997). Remember that? A comparison of real-time versus retrospective recall of smoking lapses. *Journal of Consulting and Clinical Psychology, 65*, 292–300.

Shiffman, S., Paty, J. A., Gnys, M., Kassel, J. A., & Hickcox, M. (1996). First lapses to smoking: Within-subjects analysis of real-time reports. *Journal of Consulting and Clinical Psychology, 64*, 366–379.

Shiffman, S., & Stone, A. A. (1998). Introduction to the special section: Ecological momentary assessment in health psychology. *Health Psychology, 17*, 3–5.

Shiffman, S., & Waters, A. J. (2004). Negative affect and smoking lapses: A prospective analysis. *Journal of Consulting and Clinical Psychology, 72*, 192–201.

Siegal, H. A., Li, L., & Rapp, R. C. (2002). Case management as a therapeutic enhancement: Impact on post-treatment criminality. *Journal of Addictive Diseases, 21,* 37–46.

Silverman, K., Robles, E., Mudric, T., Bigelow, G. E., & Stitzer, M. L. (2004). A randomized trial of long-term reinforcement of cocaine abstinence in methadone-maintained patients who inject drugs. *Journal of Consulting and Clinical Psychology, 72,* 839–854.

Silverman, K., Svikis, D., Wong, C. J., Hampton, J., Stitzer, M. L., & Bigelow, G. E. (2002). A reinforcement-based therapeutic workplace for the treatment of drug abuse: Three-year abstinence outcomes. *Experimental and Clinical Psychopharmacology, 10,* 228–240.

Simpson, D. D. (2004). A conceptual framework for drug treatment process and outcomes. *Journal of Substance Abuse Treatment, 27,* 99–121.

Simpson, D. D., Joe, G. W., & Broome, K. M. (2002). A national 5-year follow-up of treatment outcomes for cocaine dependence. *Archives of General Psychiatry, 59,* 538–544.

Simpson, T. L., Kivlahan, D. R., Bush, K. R., & McFall, M. E. (2005). Telephone self-monitoring among alcohol use disorder patients in early recovery: A randomized study of feasibility and measurement reactivity. *Drug and Alcohol Dependence, 79,* 241–250.

Sinha, R. (2001). How does stress increase risk of drug abuse and relapse? *Psychopharmacology, 158,* 343–359.

Sinha, R., Catapano, D., & O'Malley, S. (1999). Stress-induced craving and stress response in cocaine dependent individuals. *Psychopharmacology, 142,* 343–351.

Sinha, R., Talih, M., Malison, R., Cooney, N., Anderson, G. M., & Kreek, M. J. (2003). Hypothalamic-pituitary-adrenal axis and sympatho-adreno-medullary responses during stress-induced and drug cue-induced cocaine craving states. *Psychopharmacology, 170,* 62–72.

Sobell, L. C., Ellingstad, T., & Sobell, M. B. (2000). Natural recovery from alcohol and drug problems: Methodological review of the research with suggestions for future directions. *Addiction, 95,* 749–764.

Sobell, L. C., Maisto, S. A., Sobell, M. B., & Cooper, A. M. (1979). Reliability of alcohol abusers' self-reports of drinking behaviors. *Behavior Research Therapy, 17,* 157–160.

Sobell, L. C., Sobell, M. B., Toneatto, T., & Leo, G. I. (1993). What triggers the resolution of alcohol problems without treatment? *Alcoholism: Clinical and Experimental Research, 17,* 217–224.

Sobell, M. B., & Sobell, L. C. (2000). Stepped care as a heuristic approach to the treatment of alcohol problems. *Journal of Consulting and Clinical Psychology, 68,* 573–579.

Sofuoglu, M., & Kosten, T. R. (2006). Emerging pharmacological strategies in the fight against cocaine addiction. *Expert Opinion on Emerging Drugs, 11,* 91–98.

Stevens, S. E., Hynan, M. T., & Allen, M. (2000). A meta-analysis of common factor and specific treatment effects across the outcome domains of the phase model of psychotherapy. *Clinical Psychology: Science and Practice, 7*, 273–290.

Stout, R. L., Rubin, A., Zwick, W., Zywiak, W., & Bellino, L. (1999). Optimizing the cost-effectiveness of alcohol treatment: A rationale for extended case monitoring. *Addictive Behaviors, 24*, 17–35.

Strecher, V. J., Marcus, A., Bishop, K., Fleisher, L., Stengle, W., Levinson, A., et al. (2005). A randomized controlled trial of multiple tailored messages for smoking cessation among callers to the cancer information service. *Journal of Health Communications, 10*, 105–118.

Substance Abuse and Mental Health Services Administration. (2002). *National Survey of Substance Abuse Treatment (NSSAT): Data for 2000 and 2001* (DHHS Publication No. SMA 98-3176). Washington, DC: U.S. Government Printing Office.

Substance Abuse and Mental Health Services Administration, Office of Applied Studies. (2008). *Treatment Episode Data Set (TEDS): 2005. Discharges from substance abuse treatment services* (DASIS Series S-41; DHHS Publication No. (SMA) 08-4314). Rockville, MD: U.S. Department of Health and Human Services.

Svikis, D. S., Lee, J. H., Haug, N. A. & Stitzer, M. L. (1997). Attendance incentives for outpatient treatment: Effects in methadone- and nonmethadone-maintained pregnant drug-dependent women. *Drug & Alcohol Dependence, 48*, 33–41.

Ten Have, T. R., Joffe, M., & Cary, M. (2003). Causal logistic models for noncompliance under randomized treatment with univariate binary response. *Statistics in Medicine, 22*, 1255–1284.

Tennes, K., & Kreye, M. (1985). Children's adrenocortical responses to classroom activities and tests in elementary school. *Psychosomatic Medicine, 47*, 451–460.

Tennes, K., Kreye, M., Avitable, N., & Wells, R. (1986). Behavioral correlates of excreted catecholamines and cortisol in second- grade children. *Journal of the American Academy of Child Psychiatry, 25*, 764–770.

Tiet, Q. Q., Ilgen, M. A., Byrnes, H. F., Harris, A. H. S., & Finney, J. W. (2007). Treatment setting and baseline substance use severity interact to predict patients' outcomes. *Addiction, 102*, 432–440.

Timko, C., DeBenedetti, A., & Billow R. (2006). Intensive referral to 12-step self-help groups and 6-month substance use disorder outcomes. *Addiction, 101*, 678–688.

Timko, C., & Sempel, J. M. (2004). Short-term outcomes of matching dual diagnosis patients' symptom severity to treatment intensity. *Journal of Substance Abuse Treatment, 26*, 209–218.

Tims, F. M., Leukefeld, C. G., & Platt, J. J. (Eds.). (2001). *Relapse and recovery in addictions*. New Haven, CT: Yale University Press.

Tonigan, J. S., Connors, G. J., & Miller, W. R. (2003). Participation and involvement in alcoholics anonymous. In T. F. Babor & F. K. Del Boca (Eds.), *Treatment matching in alcoholism* (pp. 184–204). New York: Cambridge University Press.

Tonigan, J. S., Toscova, R., & Miller, W. R. (1996). Meta-analysis of the literature on Alcoholics Anonymous: Sample and study characteristics moderate findings. *Journal of Studies on Alcohol, 57,* 65–72.

Trivedi, M. H., Fava, M., Wisniewski, S. R., Thase, M., Quitkin, F., Warden, D., et al. (2006). Medication augmentation after the failure of SSRIs for depression. *New England Journal of Medicine, 354,* 1243–1252.

Tsogia, D., Copoello, A., & Orford, J. (2001). Entering treatment for substance misuse: A review of the literature. *Journal of Mental Health, 10,* 481–499.

Tucker, J. A., Vuchinich, R. E., & Rippens, P. D. (2004). A factor analytic study of influences on patterns of help-seeking among treated and untreated alcohol dependent persons. *Journal of Substance Abuse Treatment, 26,* 237–242.

Vaillant, G. E. (1998). Natural history of addiction and pathways to recovery. In A. W. Graham & T. Schultz (Eds.), *Principles of addiction medicine* (2nd ed., pp. 295–308). Chicago: University of Chicago Press.

Vaillant, G. E. (2003). A 60-year follow-up of alcoholic men. *Addiction, 98,* 1043–1051.

Vaillant, G. E., Clark, W., Cyrus, C., Milofsky, E. S., Kopp, J., Wulsin, V. W., et al. (1983). Prospective study of alcoholism treatment: Eight year follow-up. *American Journal of Medicine, 75,* 455–463.

Van Straten, A., Tiemens, B., Hakkaart, L., Nolen, W. A., & Donker, M. C. H. (2006). Stepped care vs. matched care for mood and anxiety disorders: A randomized trial in routine practice. *Acta Psychiatrica Scandinavica, 113,* 468–476.

Vanyukov, M. M., Moss, H. B., Plail, J. A., Blackson, T., Mezzich, A. C., & Tarter, R. E. (1993). Antisocial symptoms in preadolescent boys and their parents: Associations with cortisol. *Psychiatric Research, 46,* 9–17.

Volkow, N. D., Chang, L., Wang, G. J., Fowler, J. S., Franceschi, D., Sedler, M., et al. (2001). Loss of dopamine transporters in methamphetamine abusers recovers with protracted abstinence. *Journal of Neuroscience, 21,* 9414–9418.

Wagner, E. H., Austin, B. T., Davis, C., Hindmarsh, M., Schaefer, J., & Bonomi, A. (2001). Improving chronic illness care: Translating evidence into action. *Health Affairs, 20,* 64–78.

Waldron, H. B., Miller, W. R., & Tonigan, J. S. (2001). Client anger as a predictor of differential response to treatment. In R. W. Longabaugh & P. W. Wirtz (Eds.), *Project MATCH hypotheses: Results and causal chain analyses* (Project MATCH monograph series; pp. 134–148). Bethesda, MD: National Institute on Alcohol Abuse and Alcoholism.

Wampold, B. E. (2001). *The great psychotherapy debate: Models, methods, and findings.* Mahwah, NJ: Erlbaum.

Wampold, B. E. (2005). Establishing specificity in psychotherapy scientifically: Design and evidence issues. *Clinical Psychology: Science and Practice, 12,* 194–197.

Wang, G. J., Volkow, N. D., Chang, L., Miller, E., Sedler, M., Hitzemann, R., et al. (2004). Partial recovery of brain metabolism in methamphetamine abusers after protracted abstinence. *The American Journal of Psychiatry, 161,* 242–248.

Warren, K., Hawkins, R. C., & Sprott, J. C. (2003). Substance abuse as a dynamical disease: Evidence and clinical implications of nonlinearity in a time series of daily alcohol consumption. *Addictive Behaviors, 28,* 369–374.

Waters, A. J., Shiffman, S., Bradley, B. P., & Mogg, K. (2003). Attentional shifts to smoking cues in smokers. *Addiction, 98,* 1409–1417.

Weisner, C., Delucchi, K., Matzger, H., & Schmidt, L. (2003). The role of community services and informal support on five-year drinking trajectories of alcohol dependent and problem drinkers. *Journal of Studies on Alcohol, 64,* 862–873.

Weisner, C., Mertens, J., Parthasarathy, S., Moore, C., Hunkeler, E. M., Hu, T., et al. (2000). The outcome and cost of alcohol and drug treatment in an HMO: Day hospital versus traditional outpatient regimens. *Health Services Research, 35,* 791–812.

Weisner, C., Mertens, J., Parthasarathy, S., Moore, C., & Lu, Y. (2001). Integrating primary medical care with addictions treatment: A randomized controlled trial. *JAMA, 286,* 1715–1723.

West, R. (2007). Clinical significance of "small" effects of smoking cessation treatments. *Addiction, 102,* 506–509.

White, W. L. (1998). *Slaying the dragon: The history of addiction treatment and recovery in America.* Bloomington, IL: Chestnut Health Systems.

White, W. L. (2007). The new recovery advocacy movement in America. *Addiction, 102,* 696–703.

White, W. L. (2008). *Recovery management and recovery-oriented systems of care: Scientific rationale and promising practices.* Pittsburgh, PA: Northeast Addiction Technology Center.

White, W. L. (2009). The mobilization of community resources to support long-term addiction recovery. *Journal of Substance Abuse Treatment, 36,* 146–158.

White, W. L., & Kurtz, E. (2006). *Recovery.* Pittsburgh, PA: Institute for Research, Education, and Training in Addictions.

Willenbring, M. L., & Olson, D. H. (1999). A randomized trial of integrated outpatient treatment for medically ill alcoholic men. *Archives of Internal Medicine, 159,* 1946–1952.

Wilson, G. T., Vitousek, K. M, & Loeb, K. L. (2000). Stepped care treatment for eating disorders. *Journal of Consulting and Clinical Psychology, 68,* 564–572.

Witbrodt, J., Bond, J., Kaskutas, L. A., Weisner, C., Jaeger, G., Pating, D., & Moore, C. (2007). Day hospital and residential addiction treatment: Randomized and nonrandomized managed care clients. *Journal of Consulting and Clinical Psychology, 75,* 947–959.

Witkiewitz, K., & Marlatt, G. A. (2004). Relapse prevention for alcohol and drug problems: That was Zen, this is Tao. *American Psychologist, 59,* 224–235.

Witkiewitz, K., van der Maas, H. L. J., Hufford, M. R., & Marlatt, G. A. (2007). Nonnormality and divergence in posttreatment alcohol use: Reexamining the Project MATCH data "another way." *Journal of Abnormal Psychology, 116,* 378–394.

Zaharakis, N., Courtright, L., Prasad, D., Stoeckle, J., Sorensen, L., Kampman, K., et al. (2008, June–July). *Design and implementation of an adaptive treatment trial for alcohol dependence*. Meeting of the Research Society on Alcoholism, Washington, DC.

Zarkin, G. A., Dunlap, L. J., Hicks, K. A., & Mamo, D. (2005). Benefits and costs of methadone treatment: Results from a lifetime simulation model. *Health Economics, 14,* 1133–1150.

INDEX

individualized vs. group treatment/adaptive protocols, 166
possible augmentations for nonresponders, 165
possible treatment switches for nonresponders, 165–166
MET. *See* Motivational enhancement therapy
Meta-analysis, 180
Methadone
for opiate-dependent patients, 170, 213
stepped care for, 122–123
sustained provision of, 167
Methadone maintenance (MM), 78, 87–88
Methamphetamines, 24–25, 171
Method of delivering services, 59
MI. *See* Motivational interviewing
Minnesota model, 36–37
MM. *See* Methadone maintenance
Modafinil, 177
Moderate risk, 229, 235
Monitoring
extended adaptive, 124–126
technology for, 201–202
Moral inventory, 39
MORE. *See* My Ongoing Recovery Experience
Motivated patient (vignette), 6–7
Motivation, 178, 179, 233
Motivational enhancement therapy (MET), 64, 67, 96–97
Motivational interviewing (MI), 94, 96–97, 141, 142
Multicomponent protocol, 73–74
Multimodal employee assistance program, 53
Mu-opioid receptor gene, 98
My Ongoing Recovery Experience (MORE), 202–203

NA (Narcotics Anonymous), 38
Naltrexone
adaptive algorithm for, 140–144
for alcohol dependence, 88
continuation of, 127
for opiate addiction, 170, 213
responses to, 98
Narcotics Anonymous (NA), 38
National Institute on Alcohol Abuse and Alcoholism, 42, 103
National Institute on Drug Abuse, 42
Negative affect, 28
Neighborhoods, 21

Neurocognitive processes, recovery of normal, 24–26
Neuroscience research, 22–26
biological factors in addiction/relapse vulnerability, 22–24
recovery of normal neurocognitive processes, 24–26
New York state, 193
Nicotine use, 195
Nonexperimental approaches, 108–109
Nonresponse, 183
Nortriptyline, 89
Nurse care managers, 192

OASAS (Office of Alcoholism and Substance Abuse Services), 193
OCM (outreach case management), 71
Office of Alcoholism and Substance Abuse Services (OASAS), 193
Ondansetron, 179
OP (standard outpatient care), 41
Opiate addiction, 167
Opiate dependence, 123–124, 170, 213
Opioid system, 98
Orbitofrontal cortex, 22
Orientation sessions, 73, 225–227
Oslin, David, 140, 142, 143, 195
Outcome measure approach (to tailoring variables), 158–159
Outpatient care
integrated, 86–87
intensive. *See* Intensive outpatient programs
standard, 41
as traditional approach, 37–38
Outreach, active, 71, 209–210
Outreach case management (OCM), 71

Passive referral (PR), 71
Patient-by-treatment matching, 13, 94–99
genetics-based, 98–99
level of care (matching), 94–96
type of behavioral treatment, 96–98
Patient-centered care, 192
Patient choice
in adaptive algorithms, 111–112
evaluating interventions with, 187
12-step programs vs., 200
Patient education, 178
Patient Placement Criteria (ASAM), 94–95, 108
Patient preference

improving adaptive algorithms with, 215

role of, 169–170

study of, 177

understanding, 216

Patients (term), 15

Patient with barriers to participation in ongoing treatment (vignette), 8

Peer-staffed recovery centers, 200–201

Peer support, 199

Persistence, 178

Personal health, 159

Personal telephone calls, 73

Pharmacological treatments, extended, 87–89

Pharmacotherapy algorithm for alcoholism, 140–144

Philadelphia, Pennsylvania, 218

Philadelphia VAMC, 195–196

Physician health programs (PHPs), 84–85

Physicians, addicted, 84–85

Powerlessness, admitting, 38

PR (passive referral), 71

"Practice Guidelines for Recovery-Oriented Behavioral Health Care" (Connecticut Department of Mental Health and Addictions Services), 200

Pretreatment groups, 176–177

Primary care, 195–197, 218–219

Primary hypotheses, 111

Prioritization, of counseling, 232–233

Problem drinkers, 122

Problem solving, 233

Professionals, addicted, 84–85

Progress assessment, 228–231

Progress Assessment Worksheet, 226

Progress review, 232

Project MATCH, 42, 66–67, 75, 96, 97, 103, 198

Protective factors, 28–30, 231

Proximal relapse triggers, 20

Psychiatric disorders, 21

Psychiatric severity, 95–96

Psychosocial factors (of relapse), 20–22

Psychotherapeutic treatment options, 179–180

Public health and safety, 159

Quality improvement, 169, 192–193

Quasi-experimental studies

of continuing care, 44–45

of retention, 68–69

Randomization

algorithm with, 181–182

in experimental designs, 109

multiple, 183–184

sequential, 111, 215

Randomized two-group comparison, 184–185

Rates of participation in study, 60

Rational Recovery, 40

Recovery coaching, 194–195, 211

Recovery houses, 197

Recovery management checkups (RMC), 125–126

Recovery monitoring, 159

Recovery-oriented models, 198–201

Recovery Support Services, 194

Recovery Training and Self-Help, 52–53

Rehearsing new coping behaviors, 147

Relapse

biological factors in, 22–24

cognitive–behavioral model of, 26–27

immediate antecedents of, 26–28

psychosocial factors associated with, 20–22

vulnerability to, 20

Relapse prevention (RP), 56, 64–65, 128–129

Resistance to treatment, 195

Retention, 176–179

and attractiveness of treatment, 176–178

improving, 214

and incentives, 178

and persistence/advanced directives, 178–179

Retention research, 68–74

correlational/quasi-experimental studies, 68–69

experimental, 69–74

Revia, 170

Reward learning processes, 23

Risk factors, 30, 230

Risk stratification, 192

RMC. See Recovery management checkups

RP. See Relapse prevention

Scheduling phone calls, 234

Scott, Chris, 178

Secondary hypotheses, 111

Self-determination, 199, 220

Self-efficacy, 21, 28

Self-help

in alcohol care management, 195

ABOUT THE AUTHOR

James R. McKay, PhD, is a professor of psychology in psychiatry at the University of Pennsylvania. He is the director of the Penn Center on the Continuum of Care in the Addictions and the director of the Philadelphia Veterans Affairs Center of Excellence in Substance Abuse Treatment and Education. Dr. McKay received a doctorate from Harvard University. He completed a clinical psychology internship at McLean Hospital and a postdoctoral fellowship in treatment outcome research at Brown University. He is the recipient of a K02 Independent Scientist Award from the National Institute on Drug Abuse (NIDA), as well as numerous research grants from NIDA and the National Institute on Alcohol Abuse and Alcoholism, including a P01 Center on Adaptive Treatment for Alcoholism. Dr. McKay has published widely on the development and evaluation of continuing care interventions for alcohol and cocaine use disorders. His most recent work has focused on adaptive approaches to the long-term management of substance use disorders and the degree to which patients' treatment preferences influence retention and outcome.

277